Introduction To
MODERN
EPIDEMIOLOGY

Introduction To
MODERN
EPIDEMIOLOGY

Second Edition

ANDERS AHLBOM, Ph.D.
STAFFAN NORELL, M.D., Ph.D.
National Institute of Environmental Medicine
Stockholm, Sweden

Epidemiology Resources Inc.
1990

Library of Congress Cataloging-in-Publication Data:

Ahlbom, Anders.
    [Grunderna i epidemiologi. English]
    Introduction to modern epidemiology / Anders Ahlbom, Staffan
    Norell.—2nd ed.
       p.   cm.
    Translation of: Grunderna i epidemiologi.
    Includes bibliographical references.
    Includes index.
    ISBN 0-917227-06-9
    1. Epidemiology.   I. Norell, Staffan. II. Title.
  RA651.A6613   1990
  614.4—dc20
  DNLM/DLCL   90-3243

Epidemiology Resources Inc.
P.O. Box 57
Chestnut Hill, MA 02167

Translated from Swedish by Gunilla Ahlbom.

Cover Design: Sylvia Steiner

Printed in the United States of America

Table of Contents

Foreword

An old joke had it that an epidemiologist was a physician who could count. Nowadays epidemiology has changed; no longer the province of a few dedicated physicians, it has evolved into a distinct research discipline. Like many other disciplines, epidemiology demands of its aspiring students years of advanced training if state-of-the-art proficiency is to be achieved. During the past 20 years, the principles that underlie the conduct and interpretation of epidemiologic research have developed rapidly from a set of loosely understood common-sense rules of thumb into a body of logically related formal concepts that offer a coherent theory to guide the planning and interpretation of epidemiologic work. Whereas intuition and experience formerly dominated epidemiologic thinking, now a more clearly defined set of principles has been crystallized. These principles can steer the epidemiologist through the tangled problems of research with human populations. Common sense and experience may still be reliable resources for a researcher, but science progresses by formalizing understanding. In this regard the progress of epidemiology over the last two decades has been remarkable.

What is seen clearly to be common sense by experienced scientists may not be perceived in the same way by those new to a field. Students who inherit a set of formal ideas as the foundation for learning have the privilege of developing an advanced understanding of concepts without needing to repeat the mistakes of others. Unfortunately, many of the concepts of modern epidemiology have not, until recently, found their way into introductory books.

The publication in 1984 of this lucid monograph by Anders Ahlbom and Staffan Norell corrected that deficiency. Here, clearly put forth, are the core ideas that a beginner to the field will encounter and need to master. The presentation of newer concepts has been smoothly woven into the existing dogma, enabling a deeper level of understanding for the reader than was previously possible at the introductory level. For example, when I first studied epidemiology, my classmates and I were taught to distinguish between incidence and prevalence, but we never heard about the fundamental distinction between the two types of incidence measures, incidence rate and cumulative incidence. The use of stratification in data analysis to control confounding was presented to us then only in an advanced course. In this small volume, Ahlbom and Norell have put forth for the first time at the introductory level a clear description of these and related concepts.

i

Counting is still important in epidemiology, but understanding and interpreting the epidemiologic studies appearing in today's medical and public-health journals require a bit more. This new edition preserves the clarity and conciseness of the first edition. The biggest changes are in the chapters on study design, the basic principles of data analysis, and stratified data analysis. These topics have been expanded in keeping with the notion that a clear understanding of methods to control confounding in the analysis of epidemiologic data is essential even for an introductory grasp of epidemiologic research principles. The revised text remains true to its original purpose — a concise description of the core ideas underlying epidemiologic research. It will be a valuable springboard as well as a useful reference for those who desire to acquaint themselves with modern epidemiology.

Kenneth J. Rothman
Editor, **Epidemiology**
February 1990

Preface

This introductory text covers material that was developed, for the most part, during the last two decades. To a large extent this development was inspired by the work of the Department of Epidemiology of the Harvard School of Public Health. Although many of the building blocks were at hand already, we believe that the conceptual framework became much better defined in the course of that work, and also that a consistent theoretical framework and methodological structure was created that had not been available before. In our view it seems justified to refer to the theoretical and methodological system so developed as a new paradigm replacing the "person, place and time" paradigm.

This textbook was first published in Swedish; in Sweden it has been used mainly in medical schools, but also in some other introductory classes. The book has been well received by reviewers and students who appreciated our attempt at a concise and precise format.

We discussed the ideas behind the book with Kenneth Rothman and Nancy Dreyer, who told us that there was a niche for this kind of text in English as well as Swedish, and they suggested that the book be translated. We have enjoyed working on this project and we are grateful to Drs. Rothman and Dreyer for their encouragement and support during the process; without them this book would never have been published.

Anders Ahlbom
Staffan Norell
Stockholm
February, 1984

Preface to the Second Edition

After only five years it has become clear that this text needs revision, a result, at least in part, of the continuing rapid development of epidemiologic theory. That development together with a growing concern about public health continues to make epidemiology a highly interesting and challenging area.

The first six chapters of the book have undergone smaller, cosmetic changes, while the last chapters, on study design and data analysis, have seen major face lifts. In the study design chapters the changes reflect an increasing comprehension of the similarities rather than the differences between the cohort and the case-control study. In the data analysis chapters the development of personal computers and epidemiologic software has been important for the new text.

As with the previous edition we wish to thank Nancy Dreyer and Kenneth Rothman for encouragement and valuable criticism. We are also in debt to Sander Greenland for extensive and constructive criticism and to Gunilla Ahlbom for translating the Swedish edition into English.

Anders Ahlbom
Staffan Norell
Stockholm
December 1989

Introduction To
MODERN
EPIDEMIOLOGY

1. What Is Epidemiology?

Epidemiology is the science of occurrence of diseases in human populations. Disease occurrence is measured and related to different characteristics of individuals or their environments. (The word epidemiology consists of the Greek words *epi* = among, *demos* = people, and *logos* = doctrine, and thus means the doctrine of what is among or happening to people.) Investigation of disease occurrence is not a new phenomenon. The development of epidemiologic theory and methods in recent decades, however, has opened new possibilities and stimulated interest within many fields of application.

For a long time the predominant interest in epidemiology was the area of infectious diseases. The occurrence of highly contagious infectious diseases varied in obvious ways, and often increased dramatically during so-called epidemics. It was found that individuals who had been in contact with sick people often became ill themselves and that those who recovered seldom got sick again. Such epidemiologic observations became the basis of theories about infectiousness and immunity—and suggested effective means to prevent diseases—even before microorganisms and antibodies were discovered. One well known example is the classic study on cholera in London that was conducted by John Snow in 1854 (Snow 1855).

Early epidemiologic observations were not limited to infectious diseases; other diseases also displayed variation in their occurrence. The distribution of different malnutritive diseases was studied early in this century and related to certain characteristics of food composition. Even before essential nutrients, such as certain vitamins, had been identified, theories about the causes of malnutritive diseases were formulated, preventive means undertaken, and sick people successfully treated. Studies on the distribution of pellagra undertaken by Goldberger between 1915 and 1926 (Terris 1964) form a good example of this process.

During the last few decades increasing attention has focused on the epidemiology of malignant diseases. Epidemiologic studies contributed decisively to understanding the role of cigarette smoking in the occurrence of lung cancer. Other studies have shown that there is an association between exposure to some types of ionizing radiation and certain forms of cancer. Many epidemiologic studies have demonstrated the connection between exposure to certain chemical substances and some kinds of malignant tumors. Although knowledge about the etiologic mechanisms for these diseases is still rudimentary, epidemiologic in-

1

vestigations occasionally have provided a sufficient lead for the implementation of preventive measures.

Another current field of application of great importance is cardiovascular disease. In this century myocardial infarction has become a leading cause of death in the industrialized world. One plausible explanation for this increase is the profound change in what has come to be known as "lifestyle." The role of various components of lifestyle is not clear, however. We still lack fundamental knowledge on the relative importance of factors such as stress, limited physical activity, smoking, high intake of calories and high proportion of saturated fats, and we do not know what the relation is between these characteristics and elevated blood pressure, serum cholesterol and triglycerides (blood fats). In recent years, a large number of epidemiologic studies have evaluated the role of these and other characteristics in causing myocardial infarction to clarify ways in which the disease can be prevented. With similar questions in mind, other vascular diseases such as stroke have also been studied.

In the past, attention has been focused mainly on diseases with short duration (e.g., acute infectious diseases), while in more recent years the focus has been increasingly on chronic diseases. Chronic diseases are of great importance because they represent longstanding suffering for many people and a considerable burden to the health-care system. An example is joint disease, such as rheumatoid arthritis. Even after corrections for differences in the age and sex distribution, substantial differences remain in the frequency of rheumatoid arthritis between different populations. Epidemiologists are now asking, "Which characteristics among the individuals (e.g., genetic) or their environment (e.g., exposure to infectious agents) explain these differences in morbidity from rheumatoid arthritis?" Another example is intestinal diseases such as ulcerative colitis and Crohn's disease. What affects the occurrence of these diseases and the risk of complications (e.g., colon cancer)? Other epidemiologic studies have focused on variations in the frequency of birth defects and the impact of factors such as smoking, alcohol consumption, drug use, and infections during pregnancy.

Sometimes the starting point for an epidemiologic study is a certain characteristic or exposure rather than a disease. In studies of occupational hazards the starting point often is a characteristic of the occupational environment or work place; the effect of the exposure can be evaluated by measuring the health status or the frequency of disease occurrence in the occupational group and comparing it with a suitable reference group. For instance, how does exposure to asbestos in certain occupations affect the occurrence of diseases such as asbestosis, mesothelioma, and lung cancer? What is the relation of irregular working hours or occupational stress to health? What are the health hazards associated with mercury pollution from industries or use of insecticides in agriculture? In studies of side-effects of drugs the starting point again is a certain characteristic (drug exposure) rather than a disease.

These examples of fields of application suggest a close connection between epidemiology and preventive medicine. Prevention programs are rarely implemented for an entire population; therefore, prevention programs may be planned to enable studies of the effect of the intervention on the disease frequency in the population by comparing disease rates among those receiving the preventive program with rates among those who do not. In this way there is usually an opportunity to evaluate preventive measures that have been undertaken, using *experimental epidemiology*.

In recent years the value of information about disease distribution for planning the delivery of health care has become more apparent. In several studies disease occurrence has been related to health-care need, demand, and supply. There is also an increasing interest in studying the effectiveness of the health-care system and/or of different treatments.

The common basis for these different applications of epidemiology is the study of disease occurrence and its relation to various characteristics of individuals or their environment.

Additional Reading

Breslow NE, Day NE: Statistical Methods in Cancer Research. Volume I—The Analysis of Case-control Studies. International Agency for Research on Cancer 1980. IARC Scientific Publications No. 32.

Breslow NE, Day NE: Statistical Methods in Cancer Research. Volume II—The Design and Analysis of Cohort Studies. International Agency for Research on Cancer 1987. IARC Scientific Publications No. 82.

Checkoway H, Neil EP, Crawford-Brown DJ: Research Methods in Occupational Epidemiology. Oxford University Press, Oxford 1989.

Greenland S (ed): Evolution of Epidemiologic Ideas: Annotated Readings on Concepts and Methods. Epidemiology Resources Inc. Chestnut Hill, 1987.

Kelsey JL, Thompson WD, Evans AS: Methods in Observational Epidemiology. Oxford University Press, Oxford 1986.

Kleinbaum DG, Kupper LL and Morgenstern H: Epidemiologic Research. Principles and Quantitative Methods. Wadsworth, Inc. 1982.

Lilienfeld AM, Lilienfeld DE: Foundations of Epidemiology. Second edition. Oxford University Press 1980.

MacMahon B, Pugh TF: Epidemiology Principles and Methods. Little, Brown and Company 1970.

Miettinen OS: Theoretical Epidemiology. John Wiley & Sons, New York 1985.

Monson RR: Occupational Epidemiology. CRC Press, Inc. 1980.

Rothman KJ: Modern Epidemiology. Little, Brown & Co, Boston 1986.

Schlesselman J: Case-control Studies. Oxford University Press 1982.

Snow J: On the mode of communication of cholera. Churchill 1855. *In*: Snow on Cholera. Commonwealth Fund 1936. Reprinted by Hafner Press 1965.

Terris M: Goldberger on Pellagra. Louisiana State University Press 1964.

2. Measures of Disease Occurrence

The previous chapter indicated that the objective of epidemiologic studies is to learn about the occurrence of diseases. Measures of disease occurrence are therefore central to all epidemiologic activity. Such measures can be formulated in a variety of ways.

Absolute numbers and numbers related to size of the population

To start with, measures of disease occurrence should generally be independent of the size of the population. To accomplish this, the number of cases of disease is related to the number of individuals in the population. For some administrative purposes the absolute number of cases may be relevant, but for most analytical purposes the size of the population that gives rise to the cases has to be taken into account.

Example: In a campaign aimed to encourage the use of life vests, some epidemiologic data were provided. Out of 125 people who drowned, only 11 used life vests, while 114 did not. These data were presumed to suggest an association between use of life vests and risk of drowning. The comparison, however, involves two absolute numbers of cases; the sizes of the two populations that gave rise to these drowning victims, those who wore life-vests and those who did not, have not been taken into account. The observed discrepancy might well reflect only that the size of the population of life-vest users is small compared with the size of the population of non-users.

Incidence and prevalence

Measures of disease occurrence can describe either the pool of existing cases, or the occurrence of new cases. Measures of **prevalence** describe what proportion of the population has the disease in question at one specific point in time. Measures of **incidence**, on the other hand, describe the frequency of occurrence of new cases during a time period. It is useful to think of each individual as being in one of two "states": diseased or disease-free. In this framework the prevalence measure describes the proportion of the population that is in the diseased state at a specific time. The incidence measure describes the rate of flow from the disease-free state to the diseased state.

The magnitude of disease prevalence obviously depends on incidence, since a greater rate of occurrence of new cases will tend to increase the number of existing cases; but it also depends on the duration of the disease. Thus, a change in prevalence may be an effect either of a change in incidence or a change in duration of the disease. The duration in turn depends upon the time it takes to get well or the survival time with the disease.

In epidemiologic studies where the aim is to explore causal theories or to evaluate effects of preventive means, the interest is focused on the rate of flow of cases from the disease-free state to the diseased state. The relevant measure of disease occurrence, therefore, is incidence. Measures of prevalence may be relevant in connection with the planning of health services or in assessing the need for medical care in a population. Occasionally, the choice between incidence or prevalence is made for pragmatic reasons. For example, studies of chronic diseases such as rheumatoid arthritis or diabetes, in which the point of transition from non-diseased to diseased occurs gradually, and the definition of disease is arbitrary, generally employ prevalence measures, whereas studies on cancer or myocardial infarction generally use incidence measures.

Three measures of disease occurrence

Three specific measures of disease occurrence will be presented. The first is a prevalence measure and the other two are incidence measures.

Prevalence:
The prevalence measure is called simply the "prevalence" (P) (other terms in use include prevalence rate and prevalence proportion). The prevalence is defined as:

$$P = \frac{\text{number of individuals having the disease at a specific time}}{\text{number of individuals in the population at that point in time}}$$

The prevalence corresponds to the proportion of the population that has the disease at a certain point in time. Like all proportions it is dimensionless and can never take values less than 0 or greater than 1.

Example: A sample including 1,038 women age 70–74 years was selected from the population of Stockholm (Allander 1970). After examination, 70 were classified as having the diagnosis of rheumatoid arthritis. The prevalence of rheumatoid arthritis was

$$P = \frac{70}{1,038} = 0.07 \text{ for women age 70–74.}$$

5

Cumulative Incidence:

The next measure to be defined is called the "cumulative incidence" (CI) (other terms are cumulative incidence rate and incidence proportion). The definition is

$$CI = \frac{\text{number of individuals who get the disease during a certain period}}{\text{number of individuals in the population at the beginning of the period}}$$

Both numerator and denominator include only those individuals who at the beginning of the period are free from the disease and therefore at risk to get it. The cumulative incidence is, therefore, the proportion of individuals in the disease-free state at the beginning of the period that move to the disease state during the period. That is, the numerator is a subset of the denominator. Simply stated, the cumulative incidence is the proportion of healthy individuals who get the disease during a certain period. Alternatively, it can be viewed as the average risk for the individuals in the population to get the disease during that period. Being a proportion, the cumulative incidence is dimensionless and can only take numeric values in the range from 0 to 1. (Occasionally the cumulative incidence is defined in a theoretical way with a slightly different numerator, namely the estimated number of individuals who would have developed the disease if no-body had died during the interval from other diseases.)

In some studies different subgroups of the study population are considered at risk of getting the disease during different periods of time and individuals are considered at risk for periods of varying lengths. This variation in the risk period derives from the fact that different individuals enter the study at different points in time or that some migrate during the observation period. In such situations the cumulative incidence may not be directly calculable from the data. The length of the observation period directly affects the cumulative incidence: the longer the period, the greater the cumulative incidence. An extreme example would be the study of total mortality among newborn infants over, say, the ensuing 115 years. The cumulative incidence would always be 100% although the timing of the deaths could vary considerably between populations. The length of the period at risk must therefore always be reported along with the cumulative incidence and taken into account in interpreting any reported value of cumulative incidence. The mortality from other, competing, causes of death also influences the cumulative incidence as defined here; some of those dying from other causes would have been expected to develop the disease under study had they not died.

Example: The Swedish census from 1960 showed there were 3,076 males age 20–64 who were employed as plastic workers. According to the Swedish Cancer Environment Registry, 11 of those workers developed brain tumors during the period 1961–1973 (National Board of Health and Welfare 1980). The cumulative incidence during the 13-year period therefore is

$$CI = \frac{11}{3,076} = 0.004$$

Incidence Rate:

The basic measure of disease occurrence is the "incidence rate" (I) (an alternative term is incidence density), which is defined as

$$I = \frac{\text{number of cases of the disease that occur in a population during a period of time}}{\text{sum for each individual in the population of the length of time at risk of getting the disease}}$$

The sum of the time periods in the denominator is often measured in years and is referred to as "person years," "person time," or "risk time." For each individual in the population the time at risk is the time during which that individual is in the study population and remains free from the disease, and therefore at risk to get it. These time periods at risk are then summed for all individuals. The rationale is that the total number of individuals who move from the disease-free state to the disease state during any period of time is the product of three factors: size of the population, the length of the time period, and the "force of morbidity" that operates on the population. It is this "force of morbidity" that the incidence rate measures. Therefore the incidence rate is obtained by dividing the number of cases by the product of the size of the population and the length of the period, which is equivalent to summing the individual periods of time for each individual in the population. By dividing the number of cases by the time at risk, the length of the observation period is taken into account. Also, individuals entering or exiting the population during the observation period because of migration, competing mortality, or any other reason are automatically accounted for. Thus, by including time at risk in the definition, the incidence rate accounts for the major drawbacks encountered with the cumulative incidence measure.

In practical situations it is often not possible to calculate the time at risk for each individual. It may not even be possible to exclude the period during which some of the individuals are no longer at risk because they already have developed the disease. An approximation to the total time at risk that is usually satisfactory can be obtained by multiplying the average of the population size at the beginning and the end of the observation period by the length of the period. The size of the population at the middle of the observation period may also be used for this approximation.

The incidence rate is not a proportion like the two previous measures, since the numerator is the number of cases and the denominator is the number of person-time units. The magnitude of the incidence rate can never be less than zero but there is no upper limit for the numerical value of the incidence rate. This property can easily be understood by considering that the value of the incidence rate would change drastically if person months were used instead of person years.

Example: In 1973 there were 29 cases of myocardial infarction in Stockholm among men age 40–44 years (Ahlbom 1978). The number of person-years was 41,532 for men in that age group. The incidence rate is therefore

$$I = \frac{29}{41,532} = 0.0007 \text{ per year}$$

The interrelation among the three measures

It was stated in the beginning of this chapter that prevalence was dependent on the incidence and the duration of disease. In a stable situation this association may be expressed as follows, where D indicates average duration of the disease:

$$P / (1 - P) = I \times D$$

The denominator on the left side of the equation reflects the part of the population that is free from the disease. It is included in the formula since only those people who are free from the disease are at risk of getting it. For rare diseases, i.e., diseases where P is low, the following approximation may be used:

$$P = I \times D$$

The cumulative incidence depends on the incidence rate and the length of the period at risk. It also is affected by mortality from diseases other than the disease studied, as stated previously. If this mortality from other diseases is disregarded the following relation applies:

$$CI = 1 - \exp(-I \times t)$$

where t is the length of the period and "exp" indicates that the mathematical constant $e \approx 2.718$ should be raised to the power given by the expression in parenthesis. For diseases with low incidence rate or when the period is short, the following approximation may be used:

$$CI = I \times t$$

Crude and specific measures

The measures of disease occurrence discussed above may be calculated for a whole population or calculated separately for parts of the population. In the first case the measures are called "crude" measures and in the latter case "specific" measures. For example, if incidence rates are calculated for different age groups within a population, they are referred to as age-specific incidence rates. A population is divided into subgroups, called strata, when there is reason to believe that the occurrence of the disease may vary from one group to another. These variations may be of interest in themselves, but remain hidden if only crude measures are assessed. The magnitude of a crude measure for a population depends not only on the magnitude of the specific measures that apply to subgroups of the population, but also on the way the population is distributed over the different subpopulations.

Example: One year the crude mortality rate (number of deaths divided by the mean population size during the year) in Sweden was 0.010 per year while in Costa Rica it was only 0.008 per year. The explanation for the difference was not that it was riskier to live in Sweden than in Costa Rica. All age-specific mortality rates, except those for the oldest age category, were higher in Costa Rica than in Sweden. The explanation is that a greater proportion of the Swedish population was in the older age categories where the age-specific mortality rates are higher.

Additional Reading

Ahlbom A: Acute myocardial infarction in Stockholm—A medical information system as an epidemiological tool. International Journal of Epidemiology 1978; 7–271–276.

Allander E: A population survey of rheumatoid arthritis. Acta Rheumatologica Scandinavica 1970; Supplementum 15.

Elandt-Johnson RC: Definition of rates: Some remarks on their use and misuse. American Journal of Epidemiology 1980; 102:267–271.

Freeman J and Hutchinson GB: Prevalence, incidence, and duration. American Journal of Epidemiology 1980; 112:707–723.

Morgenstern H, Kleinbaum DG and Kupper LL: Measures of disease incidence used in epidemiologic research. International Journal of Epidemiology 1980; 9:97–104.

National Board of Health and Welfare, Committee for the Cancer Environment Registry in Collaboration with The National Bureau of Statistics and The Swedish Work Environmental fund: The Swedish Cancer-Environment Registry 1961–73; Stockholm 1980.

Exercises—Chapter 2

1. During the period 1930–70 the annual number of deaths due to cancer in the United States increased from 118,000 to 331,000, i.e., an increase of 180%. One explanation for this steep increase in the number of cancer deaths could be an increased exposure of the population to carcinogenic substances. Name several other possible explanations.

2. When studying the relation between diet and disease, for example, morbidity can be expressed in absolute numbers (the number of cases of affected individuals) or in relative numbers (numbers related to the size of the population). Which is preferable? Explain.

3. Disease occurrence can be measured as prevalence or incidence. Which measure is better suited for the evaluation of preventive programs? Explain.

4. a) The prevalence of a disease in a population is 0.02. Explain the meaning of this in your own words.

   b) The incidence rate of a disease in a population is 5×10^{-4} per year. Explain the meaning of this in your own words.

5. Given a population with a stable age distribution, how can one explain that the prevalence of a disease is decreasing despite a constant incidence rate?

6. What is the difference between incidence rate and cumulative incidence?

7. Make up a numerical example with a one-year observation period in which the incidence rate is more than 1 per year. What will the cumulative incidence be in your example?

8. During a 4-year period there were 532 injuries due to accidents among the personnel at certain medical laboratories. The number of employees at these laboratories was 520 at the beginning of the period and 680 at the end. Which measure of occurrence can be calculated? Calculate this.

9. In a mass screening of 1,000 65-year old men, 100 were found to have a certain disease. During the following 10-year period another 200 contracted this disease. Which measure(s) of disease occurrence can be calculated? Calculate this/these.

10. Among those admitted to a psychiatric treatment center there were carriers of hepatitis B in some wards but not in others. To investigate the extent to which this affected the occurrence of hepatitis B among personnel, employees of the treatment center were examined with regard

to the presence of serological markers. Of 67 people working on the wards with carriers, 14 had markers for hepatitis B. Of 72 people working on the other wards, 4 had these markers. Which measure of occurrence of markers can be calculated? Calculate this for each of the two personnel groups.

11. To enable early discovery and treatment of cervical cancer, regular gynecological check-ups were carried out on women age 30–59 years. Follow-up of women who were found not to have the disease at the initial examination covered 338,294 person-years at risk and resulted in the identification of 123 new cases of "carcinoma in situ." Which measure of occurrence can be calculated? Calculate this.

12. In a mass screening of 5,000 women, 25 of these were found to have breast cancer. During the next five years 10 more of the examined women developed breast cancer. Which measures of disease occurrence can be calculated? Calculate these.

13. During a 5-year period 270 cases of duodenal ulcer occurred in the male population of a city. The number of men in the city was 18,500 at the beginning of the period and 21,500 at the end. Which measure of disease occurrence can be calculated? Calculate this.

14. In a study of eyesight and occurrence of certain eye diseases among 2,477 people age 52–85 years in Framingham, there were 310 with cataracts, 156 with senile macular degeneration, 67 with diabetic retinopathy, 64 with open-angle glaucoma and 22 who were blind. Which measure of occurrence can be calculated? Calculate the occurrence of the different eye diseases and of blindness.

15. During the period January 1 - December 31, 1975, there were 435 cases of bacterial meningitis within a geographical area with an average population size during the year of 7,250,000. Which measure of disease occurrence can be calculated? Calculate this.

16. According to the Swedish Cancer Register, in the years 1971, 1972 and 1973 there were 97,121 and 112 cases of pancreatic cancer, respectively, among men age 70–74 years. At the beginning of 1971 there were 309,949 men in this age group and at the end of 1973, 332,400 men. Which measure of disease occurrence can be calculated? Calculate this.

17. In an area of Washington the occurrence of multiple sclerosis (MS) was investigated among the native white population (679,478 individuals) and among those of Japanese origin (16,122 individuals). At the time of the investigation it was found that for the two groups there were 395

and 0 cases of MS, respectively. Which measure of disease occurrence can be calculated? Calculate this for each group.

18. In a suburb of Stockholm there were 21 cases of injury due to moped accidents in one year, while in a city parish with the same average population size (80,000 people) only 9 such injuries occurred (See table).

No. of injuries and person-years by age and area

Age (years)	Number of injuries		Number of person-years	
	Suburb	City	Suburb	City
15–19	20	7	4,000	1,000
20 +	1	2	76,000	79,000
Total	21	9	80,000	80,000

a) Calculate the incidence rate for the suburb and the city parish, respectively, without taking the age distribution of the two populations into account.

b) Calculate the specific incidence rate for each age group in the suburb and the city parish, respectively.

19. Of 129,600 children born in New York, 212 had spina bifida at birth. Which measure of occurrence of spina bifida can be calculated? Calculate this.

20. In a London area during the years 1970–73, 832 children were born with a birth weight of less than 2,000 g. Of these, 133 were stillborn. Of those born alive, 210 died during the first month after birth. Which measure of occurrence can be calculated for (a) stillbirth, and (b) mortality among children born alive with a birth weight under 2,000 g? Calculate these.

21. At a call of draftees in the Netherlands a screening was carried out of 19-year old men born in 1944–47 using, among other things, standardized intelligence tests. Among 405,548 men tested there were 23,360 with MMR (Mild Mental Retardation, IQ = 50–69). Which measure of occurrence of MMR can be calculated? Calculate this.

22. In a mass screening 1,329 men age 40–59 years were examined with regard to serum cholesterol and systolic blood pressure, and then followed over a 6-year period for the development of coronary heart disease (CHD). At the beginning of the period all were free from CHD (see Table).

Which measure of disease occurrence can be calculated? Calculate this for:

a) men with serum cholesterol under 220 mg/100 ml and systolic blood pressure under 147 mm Hg,

Serum cholesterol (mg/100 ml)	Systolic blood pressure (mm Hg)					
	<147		147–166		≥167	
	No. of men	No. with CHD	No. of men	No. with CHD	No. of men	No. with CHD
<220	431	10	93	3	49	7
220–259	347	19	74	6	49	6
≥260	185	19	57	11	44	11

b) men with serum cholesterol 260 mg/100 ml and higher, and systolic blood pressure under 147 mm Hg,

c) men with serum cholesterol under 220 mg/100 ml and systolic blood pressure 167 mm Hg and higher,

d) men with serum cholesterol 260 mg/100 ml and higher, and systolic blood pressure 167 mm Hg and higher.

3. Disease and Diagnosis

To describe the occurrence of disease it is necessary to decide which individuals have the disease under study. This classification is accomplished by examination of each individual with regard to symptoms, signs, and tests and by comparison of the observations with diagnostic criteria. The different diseases are included in a classification system.

Symptoms, signs, and tests

Most observations that form the basis for making diagnostic decisions can be considered to be measurements of continuous variables. The distributions of these continuous variables differ considerably among different groups. Among the patients at a primary care center or at a department of internal medicine, e.g., there are those who seek care for the clinical manifestations of diabetes (with elevated blood sugar) and those who seek care for other reasons (with usually low or "normal" blood-sugar level). In such a group of patients the disease-related variable (blood-sugar level) tends to adopt a bimodal distribution, while in the general population the distribution is unimodal. This distinction leads to considerable differences between research based on samples of the general population and research based on clinical subjects, especially when considering problems connected with accuracy of diagnosis. In principle the variables that are the basis for diagnosis may depend upon subjective observations by the patient (symptoms), subjective observations by the examiner (signs), or upon objective observations (tests).

Symptoms (sometimes called "subjective symptoms") will here refer to manifestations that only the examined person (patient) may observe, e.g., pain, nausea, or fatigue. Of course, symptoms can be perceived and described differently by different individuals and by the same individual in different situations.

Accuracy in recording symptoms is influenced by the instrument used to collect the data; standardized interview and questionnaire methods have been developed to increase reproducibility. Reporting of symptoms in interview studies, however, is affected not only by the phrasing of the questions, but also by the interviewer and the interview situation. In one survey, for example, individuals were interviewed both by physicians and by interviewers at the Swedish National Bureau of Statistics (Johansson et al. 1969). In both instances the same questions were asked regarding the presence of certain symptoms, but with different results (see Table 3.1). Further information about methodology and methodological problems in health interviews is available from review articles and textbooks (US Department of Health, Education and Welfare 1977; Bennet & Ritchie 1975).

Table 3.1

Comparison between interviews performed by physicians and by interviewers at the National Central Bureau of Statistics (NCBS) regarding the presence of certain symptoms.

NCBS-interview	Physician Interview								
	Headache			Dizziness			Fatigue		
	No	Light	Severe	No	Light	Severe	No	Light	Severe
No	19	4	0	33	6	2	33	3	0
Light	6	13	1	1	1	0	1	5	1
Severe	0	3	0	0	3	0	2	0	1

Source: Johansson et al. (1969)

Signs will here refer to manifestations that may be observed by an examiner (usually a physician), for example, rash or swelling. Ascertainment of signs is affected by the subjective judgment of one (or several) examiner(s). This subjectivity applies to observations obtained by auscultation of (listening to) the heart and lungs or by palpation of (touching) the abdomen. It also applies to X-ray examinations that include an interpretation of the radiographic film, and to microscopic examinations of tissues. The accuracy of such examinations is dependent on the degree of agreement among different examiners (inter-observer variation) and between different examinations made by one examiner (intra-observer variation). In one study, two radiologists independently examined about 20,000 chest X-rays and classified them according to signs of disease (see Table 3.2, Lilienfeld & Kordan 1966). The agreement between the two examiners, expressed as the proportion of X-rays classified by both of them in the same way (the underlined figures in the table) was 65%. Similar comparisons were made between another 10 pairs of examiners, all qualified radiologists. The agreement varied between 32% and 76%. Concordant results have been obtained in other studies when comparing two observations made independently by the same examiner, e.g., at microscopic examination of tissue (Archer et al. 1966).

Using fewer categories means that a greater proportion of those examined will belong to the same category. For example, if our interest in Table 3.2 were limited to whether or not there is any sign of lung disease, including tumor, the agreement between the two examiners would be 89%. The proportion that will be classified in the same way is also influenced by the proportion of examinations showing a certain sign. For example, if each of two examiners finds the sign in 50% of the studied population, then chance alone would yield to agreement between the examiners for 50% of those examined. But if each examiner finds the sign in 10% (or 90%) of the population, chance alone would give an agreement of 82%.

Table 3.2

Comparison between independent interpretations of X-rays made by
two radiologists, A and B.

X-ray interpretation, Radiologist A	X-ray interpretation, Radiologist B					
	Tumor	Lung	Heart	Non-Sign	Negative	Sum
Tumor	61	16	1	9	8	95
Lung	70	1320	63	861	367	2681
Heart	19	151	1322	369	1880	3741
Non-Sign	25	407	43	1716	1656	3847
Negative	28	157	91	680	8475	9431
Sum	203	2051	1520	3635	12386	19795

Source: Lilienfeld and Kordan (1966)

NOTE:

The examinations resulted in interpretations classified according to:

—*tumor*

—other major *lung* disease

—*heart* disease

—*non*-significant observation

—*negative* (normal) X-ray

In many cases reproducibility can be increased, and hence the importance of this source of error in the diagnosis reduced, by standardization of the conditions under which the observations are made. The examination routines can be standardized and sometimes detailed, and standardized criteria for classification of the observations can be formulated. In some instances subjective examinations can be replaced by more reproducible methods, e.g., recording of heart sounds and murmurs with phonocardiogram. In many studies limitations in time and resources will in practice lead to the use of interviews and questionnaires to get information about signs of disease (US Department of Health, Education and Welfare 1977).

Tests will refer here to manifestations that can be read from an instrument and hence are less dependent on subjective judgments by the person examined or the examiner. For instance, chemical analyses of blood are often made by auto-chemists analyzing the blood sample and printing the results without human participation. The reproducibility of a result can be examined, e.g., by letting a laboratory make repeated analyses of one blood sample (intra-laboratory variation) and by letting different laboratories analyze the same blood sample (inter-laboratory variation). Figure 3.1 shows the serum-glucose level in one single sample according to 10 Swedish hospital laboratories, each performing 16 analyses of the same sample. The dotted line represents the serum-glucose level according to a reference method (isotope dilution-mass spectrometry) that is thought to give the true value.

Figure 3.1

Blood-sugar level in one blood sample according to 10 Swedish hospital laboratories who performed 16 analyses each of the same sample.

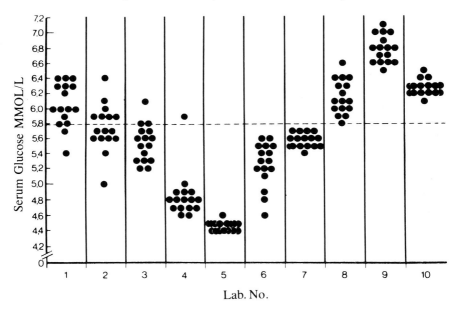

Source: Bjorkhem et al. (1981)

As seen from Figure 3.1, the inter-laboratory variation is relatively large; this variation can affect the result in epidemiologic studies where analyses have been made at different laboratories. The differences in results may be accounted for by differences in instruments, techniques, or performance. The importance of such differences has been evaluated in several studies, and the results can sometimes be used as a basis for developing procedures to decrease the inter-laboratory variation (Strommer & Eldjarn 1970; Aronsson et al. 1978).

Laboratories differ not only with respect to reproducibility of a measurement (intra-laboratory variation), but also with respect to departure from the true value. Figure 3.2 shows the results from another blood-chemical analysis (serum creatinine) where most of the laboratories show considerably higher values than does the reference method. Adjustments should be made towards the true value and not towards the mean value for different laboratories (Bjorkhem et al. 1981).

Figure 3.2

Serum creatinine in one blood sample according to 10 Swedish hospital laboratories who performed 16 analyses each of the same sample.

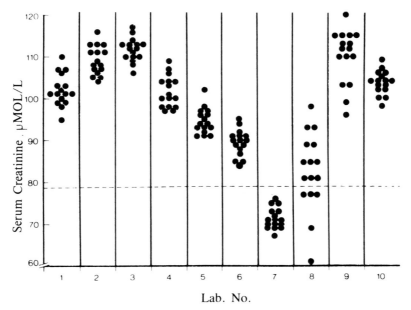

Source: Bjorkhem et al. (1981)

The variations described in Figures 3.1 and 3.2 are caused by differences in the analysis of a blood sample. In addition there are other sources of error, affecting the accuracy of a measurement, e.g., conditions when the sample was drawn (fasting, drugs, stress etc.) and the technique used to draw the blood sample. In practice it is often easier to standardize the techniques than the conditions connected with the measurement.

Diagnostic criteria

The manifestations (symptoms, signs, and tests) that are considered to be typical for a certain disease have been used to formulate diagnostic criteria, i.e., conditions that must be fulfilled for the diagnosis to be made. The choice of diagnostic criteria therefore determines whether an examined individual is to be classified as having a certain disease. If stringent criteria are used, there is only a small probability that people who do not have the disease are being classified as having it, but a relatively large probability that some people who have the disease will be classified as not having it. On the other hand, if less stringent criteria are used, the opposite type of misclassification will tend to occur: most people with the disease will be correctly classified as having it, but there is a relatively large probability that people without disease will be classified as having it.

Diagnostic criteria for myocardial infarction, for example, have been formulated in the following way (Henning & Lundman 1975)—Myocardial infarction: Any two of the three criteria a), b), or c) should be met; or criterion d) should be fulfilled:

a) Central chest pain, pulmonary edema, syncope, or shock.

b) Appearance of a pathological Q-wave and/or appearance or disappearance of a localized ST-elevation followed by a T-inversion in two or more of the twelve leads.

c) Two elevated ASAT-values, with a maximum about 24 hours after onset of symptoms, in combination with a ALAT-maximum after about 36 hours and lower than the ASAT maximum.

d) Autopsy findings of myocardial necrosis (death of heart-muscle tissue) of an age corresponding to the onset of symptoms.

The first criterion (a) is based on symptoms and on signs that the physician finds at an immediate examination. The second and third criteria (b) and (c) are based on findings from ECG-examinations and analyses of blood samples, respectively. These examinations are usually performed on patients seeking medical care among whom a myocardial infarction is suspected. The fourth criterion (d) is based on autopsy findings.

Diagnostic criteria have been formulated for other diseases in similar ways. For most diseases, however, there are no well-defined and generally accepted diagnostic criteria.

Classification of diseases

General classifications of disease usually include broad definitions for the concept "disease." For example, the list of diseases may include injuries, intoxications, and disabilities. A discussion of the concept of disease is beyond the scope of this text.

The World Health Organization (WHO) since 1948 has published several re-

19

vised versions of the International Classification of Diseases (ICD). This disease classification contains a systematic list of known and named diseases. Most of the countries that are members of the WHO use the ICD, sometimes with their own notes and supplements.

The ICD includes 17 main groups of diseases (see Table 3.3). Each group includes a great number of disease diagnoses that are assigned three-digit code numbers (see Tables 3.4 and 3.5). As indicated in Tables 3.3–3.5, the basis for disease classification in the ICD includes the causes of a disease (see Tables 3.3:1 and 3.3:17), its nature (see Tables 3.4:140–208 and 210–229) and localization (see Tables 3.3:6–10 and Table 3.5).

Table 3.3

Main groups of diseases according to the International Classification of Diseases

1 Infectious and Parasitic Diseases
2 Neoplasms
3 Endocrine, Nutritional, and Metabolic Diseases and Immune Disorders
4 Diseases of the Blood and Blood-Forming Organs
5 Mental Disorders
6 Diseases of the Nervous System and Sensory Organs
7 Diseases of the Circulatory System
8 Diseases of the Respiratory System
9 Diseases of the Digestive System
10 Diseases of the Genitourinary System
11 Complications of Pregnancy, Childbirth, and the Puerperium
12 Diseases of the Skin and Subcutaneous Tissue
13 Diseases of the Musculoskeletal System and Connective Tissue
14 Congenital Anomalies
15 Certain Conditions Originating in the Perinatal Period
16 Symptoms, Signs, and Ill-Defined Conditions
17 Injury and Poisoning

Table 3.4

Subdivision of main group 2: Tumors, according to the
International Classification of Diseases

140–195	Malignant neoplasms, stated or presumed to be primary of specified sites, except of lymphatic and hematopoietic tissue
196–198	Malignant neoplasms, stated or presumed to be secondary of specified sites
199	Malignant neoplasms, without specification of site
200–208	Malignant neoplasms, stated or presumed to be ,primary, of lymphatic and hematopoietic tissue
210–229	Benign neoplasms
230–234	Carcinoma in situ
235–238	Neoplasms of uncertain behavior
239	Neoplasms of unspecified nature

Table 3.5

Subdivision of malignant tumors of the mouth and pharynx—three-digit diagnostic codes according to the International Classification of Diseases

140 Malignant neoplasm of lip
141 Malignant neoplasm of tongue
142 Malignant neoplasm of major salivary glands
143 Malignant neoplasm of gum
144 Malignant neoplasm of floor of mouth
145 Malignant neoplasm of other and unspecified parts of mouth
146 Malignant neoplasm of oropharynx
147 Malignant neoplasm of nasopharynx
148 Malignant neoplasm of hypopharynx
149 Malignant neoplasm of other and ill defined sites within the lip, oral cavity, and pharynx

On each level in the classification system there are special headings for unclear and unspecified cases (see Tables 3.3:16, 3.4:235–239, and 3.5:145, 149). There are also many instances in which two or more similar diagnoses might apply, which may lead to possible ambiguities when classifying an individual case.

Accuracy of diagnoses

Among those individuals that have been subject to an examination, there are those who actually have a certain disease, and those who are in fact classified as having the disease, i.e., are assigned the corresponding diagnosis. This relation is illustrated by Figure 3.3.

Figure 3.3

Examples of the possible relation between those who have a disease (bold ellipse) and those who have the corresponding diagnosis (dotted ellipse).

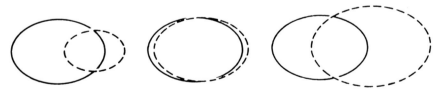

Epidemiologic data are generally based on diagnoses. When trying to judge or improve the accuracy of diagnoses the following factors should be considered:

1. Symptoms, signs, and tests:
   Results are affected by subjective judgments by the patient (symptoms) and by the examiner (signs) as well as by the accuracy of test procedures. Reproducibility can often be improved by standardized examination routines and classification schemes.

2. Diagnostic criteria:

The choice of diagnostic criteria affects the probability that individuals without the disease are classified as having it, and vice versa. For many diseases there are no well-defined diagnostic criteria.

3. Classification of diseases:

In the classification system there are adjoining diagnoses and special headings for unclear and unspecified cases on different levels. Inevitably, for some individuals it is difficult to choose among various possibilities for classification.

There is no completely accurate method to identify those individuals who have a certain disease. Some observations, though, are considered more accurate than others when making a diagnosis. One example is certain autopsy findings. For deceased individuals there is sometimes an opportunity to compare the clinical diagnosis with a more definitive diagnosis based on clinical observations together with the autopsy findings. In one study, such comparisons were made for the underlying cause of death among patients who died in a department of internal medicine at a university hospital (Britton 1974). Out of 400 consecutive deaths 383 were autopsied. The clinical diagnosis was confirmed, i.e., considered to be correct in 57%; the diagnosis was changed, i.e., considered to be incorrect in 30%. (For the remaining 13% no diagnosis was made before the autopsy.)

Naturally, diagnostic accuracy varies from one disease to another, but also from one group of individuals to another (see "Symptoms, signs, and tests" above and Chapter 4). The accuracy also depends on what kind of examination (e.g., autopsy) has been performed and on the interpretation of the observations (see 1.-3. above).

Although the objective of epidemiologic activity is the study of disease occurrence, epidemiologic studies are actually based on the occurrence of diagnoses. Lack of agreement between occurrence of diagnoses and diseases is always a potential source of error in epidemiologic research. This problem does not imply that epidemiologic studies are infeasible; but rather that knowledge of the different sources of error is essential for evaluation and improvement of the accuracy of epidemiologic studies.

Additional Reading

Archer PG, Koprowska I, McDonald JR, Naylor B, Papanicolaou GN and Umiker WO: A study of variability in the interpretation of sputum cytology slides. Cancer Research 1966; 26:2122–2144.

Aronsson T, Bjornstad P, Johansson SG, Leskinen E, Raabo E and de Verdier C-H: Inter-laboratory quality control with investigation of different methodological characteristics. Scandinavian Journal of Clinical and Laboratory Investigation 1978; 38:53–62.

Bennet AE, Ritchie K: Questionnaires in medicine. A guide to their design and use. The Nuffield Provincial Hospitals Trust 1975.

Bjorkhem I, Bergman A, Falk O, Kallner A, Lantto O, Svensson L, Akerlof E and Blomstrand R: Accuracy of some routine methods used in clinical chemistry as judged by isotope dilution-mass spectrometry. Clinical Chemistry 1981; 27:733–735.

Britton M: Diagnostic errors discovered at autopsy. Acta Medica Scandinavica 1974; 196:203–210.

Cochrane AL: Effectiveness and efficiency: Random reflections on health services. The Nuffield Provincial Hospitals Trust 1972.

Henning R and Lundman T: Swedish co-operative CCU study. A study of 2008 patients with acute myocardial infarction from twelve Swedish hospitals with coronary care unit. Acta Medica Scandinavica 1975; Supplementum 586.

Hopker WW: Das Problem der Diagnose und ihre operationale Darstellungen in her Medizin. Springer-Verlag 1977.

Johansson S, Allander E and Bygren LO: Levnadsnivaundersokningen. Metodstudie nr. 2. Jamforelser mellan lekmannaintervju och lakarintervju pa halsoavsnitt. Stencil. Sociologiska institutionen, Uppsala Universitet 1969.

Koran; LM: The reliability of clinical methods, data, and judgments. New England Journal of Medicine 1975; 293:642–646.

Lilienfeld AB and Kordan B: A study of variability in the interpretation of chest X-rays in the detection of lung cancer. Cancer Research 1966; 26:2145–2147.

Stromme JH and Eldjarn L: Surveys of the routine work of clinical chemical laboratories in 116 Scandinavian hospitals. Scandinavian Journal of Clinical and Laboratory Investigation 1970; 25:213–222.

US Department of Health, Education, and Welfare: A Summary of Studies of Interviewing Methodology. DHEW Publication 1977. No. (HRA) 77–1343, Series 2, No. 69.

Yerushalmy J: Statistical problems in assessing methods of medical diagnosis with special references to X-ray techniques. Public Health Reports 1947; 62:1432–1439.

4. Sensitivity and Specificity

Definitions

Consider a population in which some individuals suffer from a certain disease and the rest do not. Also assume that there is a method for classifying these two parts of the population, but that the method classifies some of the healthy individuals as sick and some of the sick as healthy. Healthy and sick here refer simply to absence or presence of the specific disease under consideration. Figure 4.1 illustrates the situation.

Figure 4.1

Model for sensitivity and specificity

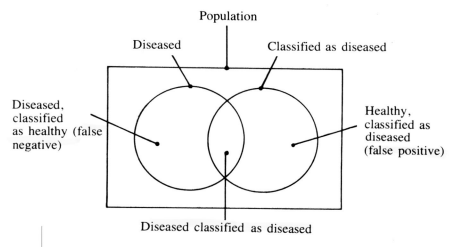

"Sensitivity" refers to the probability that a sick individual will be classified as sick and "specificity" to the probability that a healthy individual will be classified as healthy.

$$\text{sensitivity} = \frac{\text{number of sick people who are classified as sick}}{\text{total number of sick people}}$$

$$\text{specificity} = \frac{\text{number of healthy people who are classified as healthy}}{\text{total number of healthy people}}$$

Figure 4.2 illustrates schematically the interdependence of sensitivity and specificity. It is assumed that the diagnosis is based upon a measured variable for which the distributions of the sick and healthy parts of the population differ. The individuals for whom the value is above the cut-off point k of the diagnostic measure are classified as sick. If the area under each of the graphs is equal to 100%, the left part of the upper graph corresponds to the specificity, and the right part of the lower graph corresponds to the sensitivity. If the requirements for an individual to be classified as sick are made stricter, that is if k is moved to the right, the sensitivity will be decreased and the specificity increased. If the cut-off point is moved in the other direction sensitivity will increase and specificity will decrease.

Figure 4.2
The relation between sensitivity and specificity

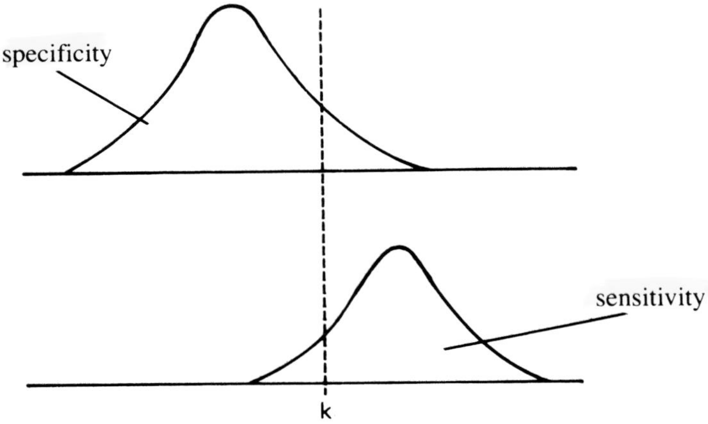

The upper curve describes the distribution among healthy individuals, the lower curve the distribution among sick individuals.

According to the figure two kinds of misclassification occur. Some of the healthy individuals will erroneously be classified as sick (false positives), while some of the sick will be classified as healthy (false negatives). The implications of these misclassifications in two different situations will be discussed.

Implications for estimation of prevalence

In studies where the aim is to estimate the prevalence of a certain disease in a population, a random sample of the population is often examined and the individuals in the sample are classified as having the disease or not. It then may seem reasonable to estimate prevalence by the proportion in the sample that is classified as having the disease. Unfortunately this procedure may result in a considerable bias.

Denote the proportion in the sample classified as having the disease by P* and as before, the prevalence by P. P* has two components. One component comes from those sick individuals that are classified as sick (true positives). The other component comes from those individuals that actually do not have the disease but erroneously have been classified as sick (false positives). The proportion of individuals that is classified as sick is then:

$$P^* = P \times \text{sensitivity} + (1 - P) \times (1 - \text{specificity})$$

and thus depends on the prevalence, the sensitivity, and the specificity. For example, if $P = 0.01$ and sensitivity = specificity = 0.99, then $P^* = 0.02$. This means that if the prevalence were estimated by the proportion that is classified as sick in the sample, the estimate would be 0.02 even though the true value is 0.01. The bias amounts to an overestimation of 100%.

The overestimation will be relatively large for small prevalences. The reason for this is that when the prevalence is low, the component in P* that comes from the healthy part of the population tends to be substantial even when the specificity is high. The healthy part of the population may be 1,000 times larger, or more, than the sick part of the population.

Since the equation above can be solved for P, a corrected estimate may be obtained in those situations where the sensitivity and the specificity are both known or may be estimated. It follows that

$$P = \frac{P^* + \text{specificity} - 1}{\text{sensitivity} + \text{specificity} - 1}$$

Example: A study of the prevalence of hypertension, defined as diastolic blood pressure above 90 mm Hg, may be used to illustrate this procedure (Rogan & Gladen 1978). In the population studied, 25% had blood pressure measurements above 90 mm Hg. From previous studies it was known that the method that was used for blood-pressure measurement had a sensitivity of 93% and a specificity of 91%. Using the above method for correction of the prevalence, a corrected value of 19% can be estimated.

Implications for screening

Another situation where false positives and negatives have to be considered is screening examinations. These examinations are intended to identify people with disease in an early enough stage that they have not yet sought medical care, in the hope that early treatment will be beneficial. The individuals for whom the screening examination gives a positive result will usually be further examined for definitive diagnosis and possible early treatment.

The proportion of those testing positive in a screening test who are true positive is called the "predictive value." The proportion testing positive is as before, $P \times$ sensitivity $+ (1 - P) \times (1 -$ specificity). The product ($P \times$ sensitivity) represents the group that is truly positive. Therefore

$$\text{predictive value} = \frac{P \times \text{sensitivity}}{P \times \text{sensitivity} + (1 - P) \times (1 - \text{specificity})}$$

Table 4.1

The predictive value for some combinations of prevalence, sensitivity and specificity

Prevalence (%)	Sensitivity (%) Specificity (%)			
	99 99	95 95	90 90	80 80
20	96.1	82.6	69.2	50.0
10	91.7	67.9	50.0	30.8
5	83.9	50.0	32.1	17.4
1	50.0	16.1	8.3	3.9
0.1	9.0	1.9	0.9	0.4

As can be seen from Table 4.1 the predictive value will be low when the prevalence is low, even for high values of the sensitivity and specificity. The predictive value is, e.g., only 50% when the prevalence is 1% and sensitivity and specificity both are 99%. This means that of those who are classified as sick by a screening test only 50% would actually be sick. The utility of a screening test depends on the cost and inconvenience for individuals and society of the additional examinations and treatments that are required and on the benefits derived from the early treatment for those who are actually diseased.

As can be seen from Table 4.1 the predictive value will be low when the prevalence is low, even for high values of the sensitivity and specificity. For example, the predictive value is only 50% when the prevalence is 1% and sensitivity and specificity both are 99%, so that of those who are classified as sick by a screening test only 50% would actually be sick. This type of misclassification must be considered in evaluating the utility of a screening test; utility also depends on the cost and inconvenience for individuals and society of the additional examinations and treatments that are required and on the benefits derived from the early treatment for those who are actually diseased.

Additional Reading

Galen RS and Gambino SR: Beyond Normality - The Predictive Value and Efficiency of Medical Diagnoses. John Wiley & Sons 1975.

Rogan WJ and Gladen B: Estimating prevalence from the results of a screening test. American Journal of Epidemiology 1978; 107:71–76.

Exercises—Chapters 3 and 4

1. As part of an epidemiologic study, 2 groups of women were interviewed about the occurrence of nausea and stomach ache. In a comparison substantial differences were found between the two groups in the reporting of these symptoms. Can the results be explained by possible differences in the method of data collection between the two groups? What are the differences.

2. To diagnose a certain disease, a method of studying cell smears under a microscope is used. The accuracy of this method is dependent on the level of agreement between different examiners. A relatively large number of samples was therefore scrutinized by two independent examiners and the result compared. Each examiner found the particular cell changes in 10% of the examined samples. The agreement, expressed as the proportion of samples that were classified alike (with or without cell changes, respectively) by the two examiners, was 80%. Is this a fairly satisfactory agreement? Why or why not?

3. In an epidemiologic study of glaucoma the examination included assessment of cup/disk ratios using the indirect ophthalmoscope. To test the reproducibility of the method two ophthalmologists examined 100 optic disks independently of each other. The findings were classified according to the cup/disk ratio. Agreement was assessed as the proportion of optic disks classified alike by the two examiners. Name three circumstances that affect the assessment of agreement.

4. Compare the problems involved in the diagnoses of cervical cancer using microscopic examination of cell smears among patients visiting a gynecologic outpatient department and among women undergoing routine gynecological check-ups, respectively.

5. At a routine mass screening of middle-aged men blood samples were taken for serum cholesterol. Of these samples, 85% were analyzed at laboratory A, 10% at laboratory B and 5% at laboratory C. Ten years later an epidemiologic study is planned where the earlier levels of cholesterol are to be related to the disease-specific mortality among these men. What is the simplest way to deal with the problem of inter-laboratory variation?

6. In several countries representative population samples have been examined to determine the occurrence of different diseases, e.g., asthma, glaucoma and schizophrenia. There are considerable differences between the findings from different countries. Can there be explanations for this other than differences in disease occurrence?

7. Give an example (other than myocardial infarction) of a disease with reasonably well-defined and generally accepted diagnostic criteria. What are these criteria?

8. The World Health Organization recommends that certain requirements should be fulfilled by those examination methods (screening methods) used in medical check-ups. According to these recommendations the methods should be safe and inexpensive and also have a high sensitivity and specificity. What is meant by (a) sensitivity, and (b) specificity?

9. A simple and inexpensive screening method has been developed to identify individuals with a specific disease at medical check-ups. To study the sensitivity and specificity the method was tested on 200 persons who underwent a simultaneous and thorough clinical examination that was considered to give an accurate diagnosis. The results are shown in the Table. Calculate the sensitivity and specificity of the screening method.

		Disease present according to screening method		
		Yes	No	Total
Disease present	Yes	60	20	80
according to	No	40	80	120
clinical	Total	100	100	
examination				

10. In a mass screening aimed at early diagnosis of a certain disease, a screening instrument is used where both the sensitivity and specificity are 99%. Of those attending the screening, one per thousand have the disease. What proportion of those who screen positive have the disease?

11. Upon what does the predictive value of a test depend?

12. Let P denote the prevalence of a disease in a population and P* the proportion of positives in a screening of that population. Suppose that the screening method's sensitivity and specificity are both 95%. Calculate P*/P for different values of P. Draw a diagram to illustrate the relation.

5. Measures for Comparisons of Disease Occurrence

In epidemiologic studies the frequency of disease occurrence among individuals who have a certain characteristic is generally compared with the corresponding frequency among those who do not have that characteristic. The compared groups are usually referred to as "exposed" and "unexposed," even when they are defined in terms of such factors as socio-economic status, serum cholesterol level, or heredity. This comparison constitutes the fundamental way of studying the association between exposure and disease occurrence. In those situations in which an association may be interpreted as causal, the comparison reflects the effect of the exposure on disease occurrence (see Chapter 6). This chapter deals with the description of the strength of the association between exposure and disease occurrence.

Absolute and relative comparisons

In comparisons of disease occurrence, the occurrence of disease is measured with one of the three measures described in Chapter 2. The comparison can be either in absolute or relative terms. Absolute comparisons are based on the difference in occurrence of disease between exposed and unexposed groups. If, for example, the cumulative incidence of lung cancer during a 15-year period is 0.0010 for smokers and 0.0001 for non-smokers, the absolute difference in cumulative incidence would be 0.0009. In contrast, relative comparisons are based on the ratio of the occurrence of disease in the exposed to the occurrence of disease in the unexposed. In the example the ratio is $0.0010/0.0001 = 10$. The numerical value will be quite different for the two types of comparative measures. The fact that the absolute measure of effect for this example is 0.0009 while the ratio measure is 10 illustrates the contrast between the numerical values.

Several arguments have been proposed to support the view that relative comparisons are more appropriate for scientific purposes. The main rationale is that the importance of a difference in disease occurrence between two populations may not be meaningfully interpreted unless related to some baseline level of occurrence. For this reason relative comparisons are more commonly used. The relative comparison measure is often referred to as a "relative risk" or "rate ratio" (RR).

Standardization

Table 5.1 describes two populations that are to be compared with respect to disease occurrence. A comparison between the two populations could be based upon the two crude incidence rates, 0.015 per year and 0.023 per year, respectively. The age distributions of the two populations differ, however. The population with the higher crude incidence rate also has the greater proportion of old people. The age distribution could be the explanation for the higher crude incidence rate in the latter population.

Table 5.1

Cases of disease and number of person-years in an exposed population and a reference population

| | Exposed Population | | | Reference Population | | |
	person-years	cases	incidence rates	person-years	cases	incidence rates
Young	3,000	30	0.010	1,000	5	0.005
Old	1,000	30	0.030	9,000	225	0.025
All	4,000	60	0.015	10,000	230	0.023

One way to improve the validity of the comparison is to perform a so-called "standardization." To understand the procedure, it is necessary to recognize that a crude rate is a weighted average of the stratum-specific rates, with weights proportional to the number of individuals or person-years in each stratum. For the exposed population in the table, for instance, the crude incidence rate is equal to

$$(3,000/4,000) \times 0.010 + (1,000/4,000) \times 0.030 = 0.015$$

To standardize for age, the crude rates are recalculated to what they would have been, had the age distributions in the two populations both been equal to the age distribution in a standard population. Suppose the exposed population and the reference population are merged to give a standard population; then 4,000/14,000 in the standard population are young and 10,000/14,000 are old. The standardized incidence rates are then:

$$(4,000/14,000) \times 0.010 + (10,000/14,000) \times 0.030 = 0.024$$
$$\text{and}$$
$$(4,000/14,000) \times 0.005 + (10,000/14,000) \times 0.025 = 0.019$$

The difference or ratio of these standardized incidence rates may be used to give an absolute or relative age-standardized comparison. The standardized incidence rate ratio (SRR or SIR), for example, is 0.024/0.019 = 1.26.

The limitation of standardization is the choice of standard population. In principle the standard population should reflect the distribution of the population for which effects are to be estimated, but it is often not clear what this means. In the above example a different standardized relative risk would have resulted if another standard population had been chosen. This method of standardization is sometimes referred to as "direct standardization."

Table 5.2 describes a common situation. For the two populations in the table, almost the same information is provided as in Table 5.1, except that for the exposed population the information on how the cases of the disease are distributed according to age is lacking. The reason for the lack of this information usually is that the number of cases is so small that a division of them into age groups would be meaningless.

Table 5.2

Cases of disease and number of person-years in an exposed population and a reference population

	Exposed Population			Reference Population		
	person-years	cases	incidence rates	person-years	cases	incidence rates
Young	3,000	?	?	1,000	5	0.005
Old	1,000	?	?	9,000	225	0.025
All	4,000	60	0.015	10,000	230	0.023

In situations like this, a comparison is often made between the observed number of cases in the exposed population (A) and the corresponding "expected" number (E). In this example A = 60. The expected number is the number of cases that would have occurred in the exposed population had all the age-specific incidence rates in the exposed population been the same as in the reference population. In this example we have

$$E = 3,000 \times 0.005 + 1,000 \times 0.025 = 40$$

For both the observed and the expected numbers of cases the underlying age distribution is that in the exposed population. The underlying incidence rates are, for the observed number, those in the exposed population, and for the expected number, those in the reference population. The ratio of the observed number of cases to the expected is therefore equivalent to a standardized relative comparison of the incidence rates in the exposed population and the reference population, with the exposed population as standard population. This method for controlling differences in age distribution is called "indirect standardization," but it should be considered a special case of the "direct" method for standardization described above. The ratio of the observed number to the expected number is often expressed as a percentage, called the "standardized morbidity (or mortality) ratio" (SMR). In the example we have:

$$SMR = (60/40) \times 100 = 150$$

Attributable proportion

In instances where an observed association can be considered to be causal, the "attributable proportion" (AP) can be meaningfully assessed (other terms in use are "attributable risk percent," "attributable fraction," and "etiologic fraction"). The attributable proportion is that proportion of the disease occurrence that would be eliminated should the exposed group have its incidence reduced to the level of the unexposed group. It is calculations of this kind that lie behind estimates that 80%, say, of all cases of cancer are attributable to the environment.

If the ratio of the incidence rate for exposed to unexposed is denoted as RR, as before, and the proportion that are exposed, among all who develop the disease, is f, we have:

$$AP = \frac{RR - 1}{RR} \times f$$

Thus, the attributable proportion takes into account the frequency of the exposure, which was not the case in absolute and relative comparisons as discussed above.

Example: In a study on the association between smoking and cancer of the mouth and pharynx, the rate ratio was estimated at 4.1 (Rothman & Keller 1972). Ninety five percent of the cases were smokers. Assuming that the observed association is causal, the attributable proportion is obtained as:

$$AP = \frac{4.1 - 1}{4.1} \times 0.95 = 0.72$$

This result means that 72% of all cases of this disease that occur in the population under study are attributable to smoking, in the sense that they would not occur if the smokers had their incidence rate reduced to the level of non-smokers. It is important to note that the result in the example is not inconsistent with an attributable proportion associated with alcohol consumption of, say, 60%. The reason that these two estimates are not incompatible is that smoking and alcohol consumption are presumed to interact in the causation of this disease. Some of the cases of mouth and pharynx cancer would not have occurred had the individuals exposed themselves to either smoking or alcohol consumption alone but not both. These cases could be prevented either by eliminating smoking or by eliminating alcohol consumption. This concept will be discussed further in the next chapter.

Comparisons based on different measures of disease occurrence

Comparisons of occurrence of disease may give different results depending on which measure of disease occurrence has been used. In Chapter 2 it was shown that the three different measures (prevalence, cumulative incidence, incidence rate) were related to one another. These interrelationships can be used to analyze how the results of comparisons depend on which measure of disease occurrence is used.

It is often preferable to use the incidence rate as the measure of disease occurrence. Therefore the incidence rate ratio (or rate difference) is often the measure of choice in comparisons of disease occurrence.

Relative comparisons of cumulative incidence give approximately the same results as do relative comparisons of incidence rates, if the period at risk is short. When the observation period is prolonged, the ratio of any two cumulative incidence measures shifts closer to unity; the ratio of two incidence rates is not affected by prolongation of the observation period.

Assuming that the prevalence of disease is low and that the duration of the disease is the same among those who are exposed and unexposed, relative comparisons of prevalence give approximately the same results as do relative comparisons of incidence rates. When the prevalence increases, however, the prevalence ratios shift toward unity. It follows, however, from the formula relating the incidence rate to the prevalence that a better approximation to the incidence rate ratio may be obtained by using the prevalence odds ratio rather than the prevalence ratio. Let subscript 0 denote the unexposed and 1 the exposed:

$$\frac{P_1/(1 - P_1)}{P_0/(1 - P_0)} = \frac{I_1 D}{I_0 D} = \frac{I_1}{I_0}$$

Therefore it is possible that the strength of an association between exposure and disease occurrence will be underestimated if comparisons are based upon prevalence or cumulative incidence, rather than incidence rates. The degree of underestimation will depend on the magnitude of the prevalences or cumulative incidences involved. Little error will occur for prevalences and cumulative incidences less than 0.1.

Additional Reading

Cole P and MacMahon B: Attributable risk percent in case-control studies. British Journal of Preventive and Social Medicine 1971; 25:242–244.

Greenland S & Robins JM: Conceptual problems in the definition and interpretation of attributable fractions. American Journal of Epidemiology 1988;128:1185–1197.

Miettinen OS: Proportion of diseases caused or prevented by a given exposure, trait or intervention. American Journal of Epidemiology 1974; 99:325–332.

Rothman KJ and Keller AZ: The effect of joint exposure to alcohol and tobacco on risk of cancer of the mouth and pharynx. Journal of Chronic Diseases 1972; 25–711–716.

6. Risk Indicators and Causes of Disease

Risk indicators

If a disease (D) is more common among those with a certain characteristic (C) than among those without it, then there is an association between C and D (Figure 6.1). If, in addition, C occurs, or is present, prior to D, individuals with C have higher risk to get the disease: C is a "risk indicator" for the disease D.

Figure 6.1

Co-variation between characteristic (C) and disease (D)

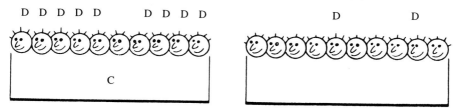

Some diseases are more common among those who live in certain geographical areas, more common among men than among women, more common in certain age groups or occupational groups, more common among smokers than among non-smokers, and so forth. Age, gender, residence, occupation, and smoking are therefore risk indicators for many diseases. Knowledge about risk indicators can be used to identify high risk populations suitable as target groups for preventive interventions or directed health check-ups.

Causes of disease

Some events or phenomena occur in a regular sequence so dependably that we can talk about cause and effect. The concept of cause has been discussed within philosophy, particularly in the theory of science (Taylor 1967). Within epidemiology causes of diseases are studied with the objective of explaining and eventually preventing the occurrence of disease. Thus, a causal association is said to exist if the disease incidence would be lower in the absence than in the presence of a specific characteristic of individuals or their environments.

A co-variation between C and D can in principle arise in three different ways (Figure 6.2):

a) C is a cause of D

b) C and D have a common cause (X), or

c) D is a cause of C.

If C occurs prior to D, then C is a risk indicator for D and only the first two alternatives (a) and (b) can apply. In the literature the term "risk factor" is often used, sometimes referring to a cause—alternative (a)—and sometimes to a risk indicator, which also includes alternative (b).

In epidemiologic studies, where the aim is to analyze possible causal relationships, it is essential to distinguish between alternatives (a), the causal explanation, and alternative (b), the "confounding" explanation.

Figure 6.2

Three explanations of co-variation between characteristic (C) and disease (D)

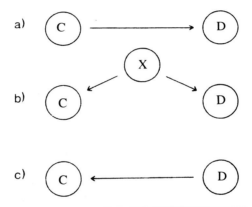

When a study result indicates a co-variation between a characteristic and a disease, two explanations in addition to (a) through (c) have to be considered: (d) inaccurate methodology (see Chapter 8) and (e) random variation (see Chapter 9).

Causal model I

A disease generally has several causes that together or separately give rise to the disease. Correspondingly, one cause can contribute to the origin of several different diseases.

Causes of disease can in principle give rise to a disease either indirectly, by activating other causes, or directly. In practice, it is almost always possible in any causal situation to think of intermediate causes. Causal relationships should therefore preferably be viewed in degrees of directness rather than as simply direct or indirect. The relationship between cause and disease can be illustrated in a model, the so called "web of causation." One example is the web of causation for myocardial infarction shown in Figure 6.3. Causes at high levels in the hierarchy, often social characteristics like food habits and stress, may be of great interest from an epidemiologic point of view and for prevention of disease.

Figure 6.3

Web of causation for myocardial infarction

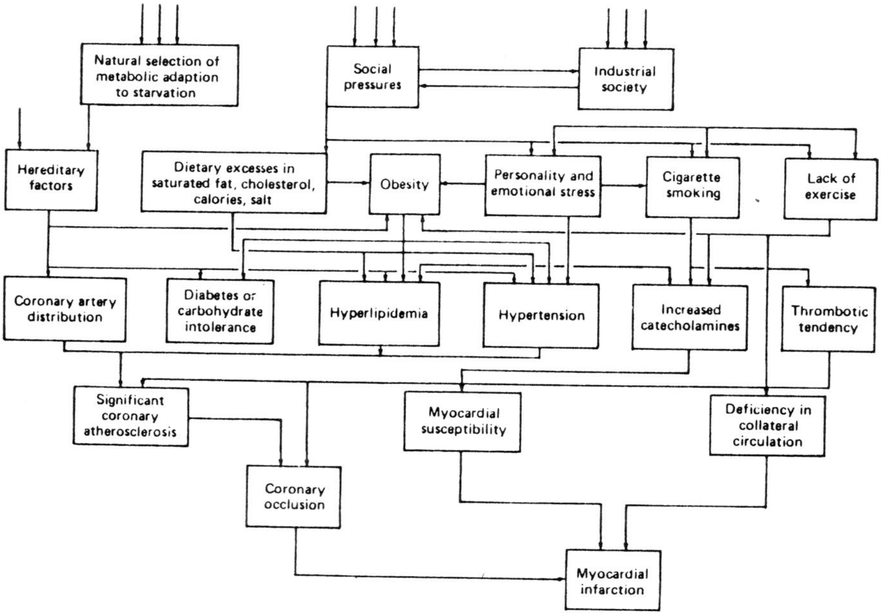

Used by permission of G. Friedman from *Primer of Epidemiology*, © 1974, McGraw-Hill, Inc.

Causal model II

A "sufficient cause" is a cause that inevitably brings a certain consequence. Single causes of diseases are rarely sufficient causes. Exposure to tubercle bacilli, for instance, does not necessarily lead to tuberculosis. The risk of developing the disease is affected, among other things, by anatomical and physiological characteristics of the individual and also by possible presence of specific immunity.

A cause that is not by itself a sufficient cause is a "contributing cause." Hyperlipidemia, hypertension, cigarette smoking, and increased thrombotic tendency, for example, are thought to contribute to the occurrence of myocardial infarction. The vast majority of all causes of disease can be regarded as contributing causes.

A "necessary" cause of disease is a cause that must be present to enable a disease to occur. Exposure to tubercle bacilli is therefore a necessary (but not sufficient) cause for tuberculosis.

The model in Figure 6.4 shows schematically how several contributing causes (sectors) together form a sufficient cause (circle). The figure also shows that a disease can have several sufficient causes and that these may have one or more contributing causes in common. A cause that, like A, is an element in all sufficient causes is a necessary cause.

Figure 6.4
Schematical description of causes of a hypothetical disease

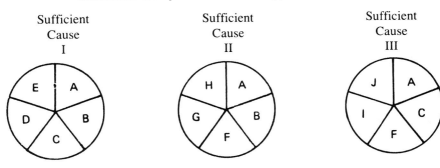

Source: Rothman (1976)

According to the model, knowledge of all contributing causes is not necessary for prevention of a disease. By eliminating one of the elements from one sufficient cause, all cases of disease that occur from this sufficient cause are prevented.

Each single cause of disease has an associated attributable proportion (AP). This measure is the proportion of all cases of the disease that is attributable to that cause; phrased in another way, the proportion of all cases of the disease that would not have occurred, had the cause been eliminated (see Chapter 5). The sum of the attributable proportions for all sufficient causes of a disease is always equal to 100%. The attributable proportion of a contributing cause is equal to the attributable proportion of the sufficient cause, or causes, in which it is an element. If, for example, AP(I) = 20% and AP(II) = 30% it follows that

AP(III) $= 100\% - 30\% - 20\% = 50\%$. The contributing causes D and E only occur in sufficient cause I where AP(D) $=$ AP(E) $=$ AP(I) $= 20\%$. The contributing causes B and A occur in two and three sufficient causes, respectively. We therefore have that AP(B) $=$ AP(I) $+$ AP(II) $= 20\% + 30\% = 50\%$ and AP(A) $=$ AP(I) $+$ AP(II) $+$ AP(III) $= 100\%$. In this example the sum of the attributable proportions for all the contributing causes, A through J, is 500%. For every disease the sum of all attributable proportions for contributing causes is 100% or more (in general much more). If, e.g., 60% of the cases of one disease are caused by smoking, 70% can very well be caused by food habits and 80% by exposure to other things. Consequently, the incidence of the disease may be reduced by up to 60% by changing smoking habits, or alternatively, by up to 70% by changing food habits, etc.

The extent to which a contributing cause participates in the development of a disease is, according to the model, dependent on the presence of the remaining elements in the corresponding sufficient cause. If, for example, the contributing cause E is present in 50% of the individuals and the combination of A + B + C + D in 40%, then the presence of E will lead to the disease among

$$\frac{50}{100} \times \frac{40}{100} = \frac{20}{100}$$

i.e., among 20% of the individuals. If E is present among 50% but the combination of A + B + C + D only among 2%, it follows that E will lead to the disease among

$$\frac{50}{100} \times \frac{2}{100} = \frac{1}{100}$$

i.e., among 1% of the individuals. (In the example it is assumed that A + B + C + D occurs independently of E.)

In a similar way it can be shown that, if the probability of occurrence of two or more contributing causes included in the same sufficient cause is increased, the effect on disease occurrence would be greater than the sum of the effects that would occur for a similar increase in the probability of occurrence of two causes included in distinct sufficient causes (so-called synergism, see exercise 21).

Additional Reading

Friedman GD: Primer of Epidemiology. McGraw-Hill, New York 1974.

Nordenfelt L, Lindahl BIB (eds): Health, Disease, and Causal Explanations in Medicine. D Riedel Publishing Co, Dordrecht 1984.

Rothman KJ: Causes. American Journal of Epidemiology 1976; 104: 587–592.

Rothman KJ (ed): Causal Inference. Epidemiology Resources Inc, Chestnut Hill 1988.

Rothman KJ, Greenland S and Walker AM: Concepts of interaction. American Journal of Epidemiology 1980; 112: 465–466.

Saracci R: Interaction and synergism. American Journal of Epidemiology 1980; 112: 465–466.

Susser M: Causal Thinking in the Health Sciences. Concepts and Strategies of Epidemiology. Oxford University Press, Oxford 1973.

Taylor R: Causation, pages 56–66 in The Encyclopedia of Philosophy, Vol 2 (ed. Edwards P). McMillan Press, 1967.

Exercises—Chapters 5 and 6

1. In a study the occurrence of respiratory cancers was determined for the male population in urban and rural areas, respectively (see below). Make relative and absolute comparisons based on the three different measures of disease occurrence.

	Urban	Rural
Incidence rate expressed per 100,000 person-years	60	15
Cumulative incidence during a 5-year period expressed per 100,000 population	315	80
Prevalence expressed per 100,000 population	275	70

2. In a study, mortality among diabetics was compared with that expected in the population as a whole. The observed number of deaths from myocardial infarction among diabetics was 1,107 and the expected number was 531. Calculate the SMR. Describe the result in your own words.

3. Of 2,872 individuals who had received radiation treatment in childhood because of enlarged thymus, 24 developed cancer of the thyroid and 52 developed benign thyroid tumors. A comparison group consisted of 5,055 children who had received no such treatment (brothers and sisters of those who had received radiation treatment). During the follow-up period none of the comparison group developed thyroid cancer, but six developed benign thyroid tumors. Calculate the relative risk for

   a) thyroid cancer, and

   b) benign thyroid tumors.

   c) Describe the results in your own words.

4. Of 725 female industrial workers exposed to radium in their work between 1915–29 in the U.S., 22 died of malignant bone tumors. The expected number was 0.27. Calculate the SMR.

5. For the data in exercise number 22 of Chapter 2, calculate the relative risk of coronary heart disease in relation to group (a) for each of the groups (b), (c) and (d).

6. Medicines used in the treatment of certain cancers are thought to increase the risk for other diseases. To study this problem, 913 women were observed who had been treated for ovarian cancer with certain alkylating agents. During the follow-up period 11 of these developed

acute non-lymphatic leukemia, compared with an expected number of 0.1. Calculate the SMR.

7. An influenza vaccine was tested on a voluntary group of young female student nurses. Of the 95 individuals who received the vaccine, 3 fell ill, and of the 48 individuals who received a placebo, 8 fell ill with influenza during the follow-up period. Moderate or marked discomfort after the "vaccination" was reported by 27% of those who received vaccine and by 24% of those who received placebo. Calculate the relative risk of

a) contracting influenza, and

b) discomfort after the vaccination.

c) Describe the results in your own words.

8. In a Finnish study of morbidity and mortality from myocardial infarction a comparison was made of married and single men. The following results were obtained:

Myocardial infarction in men 40–64 years—
(age standardized rates)

	Incidence/ 100,000 person-years	Mortality/ 100,000 person-years
Married	1,371	498
Single	1,228	683

What is the relative risk of

a) myocardial infarction for married compared with single men?

b) death from myocardial infarction for married men compared with single men?

c) How can the above results be interpreted?

9. A group (A) of 6,000 people have participated in a program for prevention of a disease. Another group (B) of 5,000 people did not participate in this program and serve as a control group. During the course of a year there were 36 cases of the disease in group A and 35 cases in group B. The result is shown in the following table, according to two age categories. Calculate the incidence rate for each of the age categories in the two groups. Make an age standardized analysis with equal weights for the two age groups, and a relative comparison of the standardized incidence rates.

	Group A		Group B	
	Number of Person-Years	Number of Cases	Number of Person-Years	Number of Cases
Younger	2,000	4	4,000	20
Older	4,000	32	1,000	15
Total	6,000	36	5,000	35

10. Among the male employees in a certain occupational group there were 40 cases of myocardial infarction in one year. The table shows the number of male employees according to age as well as the age-specific incidence rates for the male population in the country as a whole.

Age	No. Of Employees During The Year	Incidence Rate For The Country (per 1,000 person-years)
35–44	8,000	0.5
45–54	2,000	4
55–64	2,000	9

Make a relative comparison between the incidence rate of myocardial infarction among employees in the occupational group and the general population by calculating the SMR.

11. In a study, male vulcanization workers were compared with all working men with regard to the cumulative incidence of esophageal cancer during a 13-year period. The results are shown in the table below. Perform an "indirect" age standardization, i.e., calculate the SMR.

	Vulcanization Workers		Comparison Group	
Age	No. With Disease	No. Of Men	No. With Disease	No. Of Men (thousands)
15–24	?	651	0	337
25–34	?	518	6	431
35–44	?	500	90	522
45–54	?	465	381	507
55–64	?	211	626	367
Total	8	2,345	1,103	2,164

12. From the catchment areas of two local clinics, random samples were taken from the male population between the ages of 30–69. The occurrence of chronic bronchitis was studied using a previously validated questionnaire about current symptoms. The results are shown in the following tables. Perform an age standardized comparison between the two populations with equal weights for the different age groups.

Population I

Age	No. in sample	No. with chronic bronchitis
30–39	1,000	5
40–49	2,000	20
50–59	4,000	50
60–69	3,000	50
Total	10,000	125

Population II

Age	No. in sample	No. with chronic bronchitis
30–39	5,000	25
40–49	3,000	40
50–59	1,000	20
60–69	1,000	20
Total	10,000	105

13. In a suburb of Sydney, Australia, a representative sample from the adult population (20–69 years) was studied with regard to the occurrence of psychological disorders (PD) and chronic physical disease (CPD). Of the 863 individuals examined 8% had PD alone, 29% had CPD alone and 14% had both PD and CPD. Is there any correlation between PD and CPD? Why or why not?

14. a) Describe briefly the difference between risk indicators and contributing causes of disease.

b) How can knowledge about risk indicators and contributing causes respectively be utilized in the prevention of disease?

15. a) Give an example of a contributing cause, the elimination of which would lead to total cessation of the disease.

b) What is the name given to a contributing cause of this kind?

16. What is the meaning of "cause of disease" in epidemiology?

17. By abolishing the use of tobacco the incidence of a certain disease can be cut by 60%. This was interpreted to mean that 60% of the cases of this disease are caused by tobacco.

    a) What proportion of the cases of this disease are caused by factors other than tobacco (i.e., how great a proportion of the cases could be prevented by eliminating the other causes instead of tobacco)?

    b) Can any conclusions be drawn as to the relative risk of falling ill for exposed subjects (tobacco users) compared with non-exposed?

18. What is meant by the attributable proportion?

19. Explain in your own words why the sum of the attributable proportions for all causes of a disease is usually much greater than 100%.

20. Suppose that a disease has three contributing causes, A, B and C. Together they make up the only sufficient cause of the disease. In the population the distribution of A, B and C are independent of each other. A is found in 10%, B in 20% and C in 30% of the population. Calculate the proportion of the population that develops the disease.

21. Using the circumstances in the previous exercise as your point of departure, calculate the proportion of the population that develops the disease on the basis of the following alternatives:

Alternative	Occurrence (%) Of:			Disease Occurrence
	A	B	C	
0 (= previous exercise)	10	20	30	
1	10	80	30	
2	10	20	90	
3	10	80	90	

Compare the occurrence of the disease according to alternatives 1, 2, and 3, respectively, with its initial occurrence (alternative 0). Make both

a) absolute and

b) relative comparisons.

c) Describe the results in your own words.

22. What conditions determine the extent to which a contributing cause of disease affects the frequency of disease in a population? Explain.

7. Study Design

Epidemiologists use two types of study to compare incidence rates between exposed and unexposed groups. One is a "cohort study" (also known as a "follow-up" study), and the other is a "case-control" study.

Cohort studies

The cohort study is the more straightforward approach. All subjects in the study population are assigned to a category of exposure at the start of the time period under study. The exposure categorization may be dichotomous (exposed/unexposed) or it may include several categories (e.g., unexposed, low exposure, high exposure). The study subjects are then followed up for a defined observation period and all new cases of the disease under study are identified. The combination of the population and time period at risk (i.e., the person-time observed) is sometimes referred to as the study base, indicating the base experience from which the cases arise. The information obtained is used to estimate the incidence rate or cumulative incidence among the exposed and unexposed groups. The comparison of disease incidence among exposed and unexposed may be either absolute or relative. In Figure 7.1 the principle of a cohort study is illustrated.

Figure 7.1

The principle for cohort studies

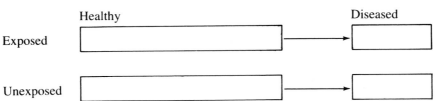

Example: The association between smoking and mortality from coronary heart disease was studied in a population of British physicians (Doll & Hill 1966). Table 7.1 shows data from that study. The age-specific incidence rates are calculated as the ratio of the number of deaths from coronary heart disease to the number of person-years at risk (in thousands). For each age group a relative as well as an absolute comparison is presented.

Table 7.1

Mortality from coronary disease among smokers and non-smokers

Age	Number of deaths per 1000 person-years		$I_1 - I_0$	I_1/I_0
	Smokers (I_1)	Non-Smokers (I_0)		
35–44	0.6	0.1	0.5	6.0
45–54	2.4	1.1	1.3	2.2
55–64	7.2	4.9	2.3	1.5
65–74	14.7	10.8	3.9	1.4
75–84	19.2	21.8	−2.6	0.9
All Ages	4.4	2.6	1.8	1.7

In **experimental** research the exposure is assigned to the study subjects by the investigator, often following a protocol that relies on a randomizing device for the assignment (as in randomized clinical trials). The purpose of random assignment is to reduce confounding. For ethical and practical reasons, however, epidemiologic investigations are usually **nonexperimental**; that is, they are based on existing exposure conditions. The unexposed group is intended to provide information about the disease incidence rate that would be expected in the exposed group if the exposure under study did not affect the occurrence of the disease. Therefore, the unexposed group should be selected in such a way that it is similar to the exposed group with regard to other risk indicators for the disease under study.

In principle there are three different approaches to defining the unexposed group:

1. Internal comparison: A single cohort is identified that contains a sufficient number of exposed and unexposed subjects.

2. External comparison: An exposed cohort is identified and efforts are made to find another cohort that is unexposed but is similar in other respects to the exposed cohort.

3. Comparison with the "general" population: An exposed cohort is identified and comparisons are made with the disease incidence in, for example, the total population of a defined geographic region (considered as "unexposed").

Confounding may occur if a risk indicator other than the studied exposure is unequally distributed between the groups (see Chapters 6 and 8). Confounding can to a certain extent be controlled in the data analysis; for example, differences in the distributions of factors such as age and sex between the groups can be corrected in the analysis. (See the section on standardization in Chapter 5, and Chapter 10.) There are other problems to be considered, however, when selecting the unexposed group.

The incidence of disease can vary considerably over time (year, season etc.), and by geographic area, ethnic background, and socio-economic status. Differences between the exposed and unexposed groups with regard to these or other factors can influence the results of the study. To avoid such problems it may be advisable to select exposed and unexposed subjects with similar distributions for these factors and to follow them during the same observation period.

There are several drawbacks in using the general population as a comparison group in cohort studies. The "healthy worker effect" (McMichael et al. 1975) describes one such problem: It alludes to a bias that results because subjects who are employed in certain occupations often constitute a group with a lower risk of developing many diseases than the population as a whole simply because the employed group must be healthy enough to work. The unemployed part of the population would therefore have a higher risk of falling ill. Thus, in a study that compares the morbidity experience of a certain occupational group with that of the total population, the healthy worker effect could lead to an underestimation of the relative morbidity among the exposed group.

If information from the total population is used to represent the "unexposed" group, then all study subjects classified as exposed (and other people with the same exposure) are also included among the "unexposed." Unless the proportion of exposed subjects in the total population is low, this dilution of the "unexposed" population may result in an underestimation of the relative morbidity in the exposed group.

The procedures used to identify new cases of the disease under study should be similar for the exposed and unexposed groups. If, for example, certain screening procedures are used to a different extent in the exposed group, case identification may be more complete in the exposed group (see Chapter 8).

Selecting more than one unexposed group can reveal to what extent the study results are influenced by the selection of an unexposed group. Separate analyses using these groups that yield similar results indicate that the results probably were not influenced by the choice of the unexposed group. Another approach that has sometimes been used to check the comparability between the exposed and unexposed group is to include comparisons of the occurrence of diseases that are not expected to be associated with the exposure under study.

Cohort studies are sometimes based on information about exposure and disease collected in the past (so called "retrospective cohort studies"). For instance, a cancer registry or cause-of-death registry is sometimes used as the source of information about cases, with considerable savings in the cost of case-finding. The accuracy of such a study depends upon the completeness of disease ascertainment in the registry for the population and time period under study. Similarly, information on "exposure" may be obtained from census data or registries providing information on certain occupational groups. Again, the savings may be substantial but the quality of exposure information should be examined before relying on such a source. In addition, information on relevant confounders may not be available from these sources.

Retrospective cohort studies are common in occupational epidemiology. Often a group of employees in an industry or factory is followed through registries recording cases of death or disease. The total population in the country or the region in question is often used as the "unexposed" group. The SMR (standardized mortality ratio - see Chapter 5) may be calculated in such studies as a measure of the effect of exposure on the rate of disease occurrence.

Example: To test the hypothesis that occupational chemical exposure increases the risk of cancer, chemical engineers graduated during the period 1931–59 from the Royal Institute of Technology in Stockholm were identified (Olin & Ahlbom 1980). This cohort was followed in the Swedish cause-of-death registry. The observed number of deaths from cancer in the cohort was 32. If the chemists in each age group had the same mortality rate as the entire working population of the country, 24.2 cancer deaths would have been expected. Therefore, the

$$SMR = 32/24.2 \times 100 = 132$$

Case-control studies

For most diseases, the occurrence of new cases is a relatively rare event. Thus, in a cohort study, a large number of study subjects may have to be examined for exposure status and followed up for a long time to obtain a sufficient number of cases. Such a study is often not practical or feasible. The problem can be avoided by using exposure information from a sample of the study population rather than including the entire study population.

Case-control studies are based on this principle. As in cohort studies, information is obtained on all cases that occur in the study population during a defined observation period. In addition, a comparison group of "controls" are selected as a representative sample of the study population; ideally the control group reflects the exposure distribution in the entire study population. Exposure information is then obtained for cases and controls only, rather than for all members of the population. Figure 7.2 illustrates the principle of a case-control study.

Figure 7.2

The principle for case-control studies

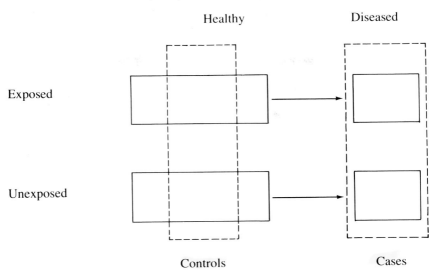

Healthy   Diseased

Exposed

Unexposed

Controls   Cases

Table 7.2

Organization of data from a case-control study

	Exposed		
	Yes	No	All
Cases	a	b	N_1
Controls	c	d	N_0

The data obtained in a case-control study may be summarized in a 2×2 table (see Table 7.2.), where N_1 and N_0 are the number of cases and controls, respectively.

Data from a case-control study can be used to estimate the relative risk (RR $= I_1/I_0$). The "odds ratio" (a/b)/(c/d) is an estimate of the relative risk (RR):

$$\frac{I_1}{I_0} = \frac{A_1/R_1}{A_0/R_0}$$

where I_1 and I_0 are the incidence rates among the exposed and unexposed, A_1 and A_0 are the numbers of cases among the exposed and unexposed, and R_1 and R_0 are the person years at risk among the exposed and unexposed. Using simple algebra, the above expression can be transformed into:

$$\frac{I_1}{I_0} = \frac{A_1/A_0}{R_1/R_0}$$

where A_1/A_0 is the ratio of exposed to unexposed among the cases (i.e., (a/b) in Table 7.2). Assuming that the controls were selected in such a way that they reflect the exposure distribution in the entire population, (c/d) is an estimate of (R_1/R_0). Thus, the odds ratio is an estimate of the relative risk:

$$RR = \frac{(a/b)}{(c/d)} = \frac{ad}{bc}$$

Example: In a case-control study of diet and pancreatic cancer (Norell et al 1986), the following data were obtained:

Table 7.3

Consumption of fried or grilled meat at least once per week among cases and controls.

	Exposed		
	Yes	No	All
Cases	53	43	96
Controls	53	85	138

Since the proportion of cases exposed is higher than the proportion of controls exposed, there appears to be an association between exposure and disease. The relative risk is estimated as follows:

$$RR = \frac{(53/43)}{(53/85)} = 1.98$$

The incidence rate is estimated to be about two times higher among the exposed (those who eat fried or grilled meat every week) than among the unexposed.

The control group in a case-control study should, as mentioned above, be selected in such a way that it reflects the exposure distribution in the study population, i.e., in the population that generated the cases. There are two different approaches to control selection:

1. A random sample of the study population. This approach has the advantage' that the controls will be representative of the study population in a formal (statistical) sense and therefore the selection process for controls does not introduce any systematic error. This option obviously requires that the population is accessible for random sampling. Potential disadvantages of random sampling for control selection are the possibility of a high non-response rate among healthy population controls, and the possibility of differences in the quality of exposure information between cases and healthy controls. (See Chapter 8, the section on misclassification.)

2. A sample of the study population that is not randomly selected. This is the only option when the cases are identified in such a way that the study popu-

lation is not accessible for random sampling. For example, if the cases are patients diagnosed with the disease being studied in a particular clinic, these patients most likely do not represent all cases of the disease occurring in a population from which a random sample may be drawn, and therefore a non-random selection of controls is necessary. Sometimes this approach is used for other reasons, such as reducing non-response among controls or improving the comparability of exposure information between cases and controls. Controls may be selected, for example, from patients who have been hospitalized (hospital controls) or who have died (dead controls) during the observation period from diseases other than the one under study. While such non-random selection schemes may result in greater comparability of cases and controls, controls selected in this way may not reflect the exposure distribution in the overall study population, thus possibly introducing a systematic error. (See Chapter 8, the section on selection bias.)

When controls are selected non-randomly, it can be difficult to judge to what extent their exposure distribution reflects the exposure distribution in the population that generated the cases. When hospital controls are selected, a single diagnostic group may be used as a source of controls, provided that neither the disease nor the probability for hospitalization is associated with the studied exposure(s). It may be useful to select two or more diagnostic groups sufficiently large to permit separate analyses to minimize the problem, especially when such associations cannot be ruled out at the beginning of the study. Using a sample of all patients (or hospitalization episodes) regardless of diagnosis is less advisable, since many exposures (such as diet, tobacco and alcohol consumption) tend to be related to several common diseases. When there is a choice between these two approaches in selecting controls, random sampling is the preferred method (Norell & Ahlbom 1987).

In case-control studies, controls are sometimes selected by individual matching to the cases: for every case, one or more controls are selected who are similar to that case in certain respects. Cases and controls are matched on potential confounders, such as age, sex and residence, for which information can be obtained before data collection begins.

The implications of matching in case-control studies are complex, and will not be further developed here. It should be pointed out, however, that matching is performed with the purpose of reducing random error rather than confounding. (Confounding can be controlled effectively by restrictions in the choice of study population and in data analysis; see the section on standardization in Chapter 5 and the section on stratification in Chapter 10). Furthermore, matching can actually introduce problems, since each case and its corresponding control(s) must be kept together during analysis.

Advantages and disadvantages of the cohort and the case-control designs

The cohort design might seem to be a more appealing choice than the case-control design. It has a simple, logical structure that leads to measurements of disease incidence for the exposed and unexposed groups, or each category of exposure if several are used. This design permits absolute as well as relative comparisons of disease incidence among the exposed and unexposed. The case-control design provides somewhat less information, in that usually only the relative risk can be estimated. Absolute measures of incidence can also be made in case-control studies, but only if the sampling fraction for the controls or the baseline incidence rate for the total study population is known. (The sampling fraction is the number of controls divided by the total number of subjects or person-years in the study population.)

Case-control studies, like cohort studies, are based on follow-up of incident cases in a certain study population during a defined observation period. Case-control studies, however, use exposure information from a sample of the study population rather than from the whole study population. Unless the disease incidence is very high, obtaining exposure information for a sample of the study population will be much less expensive and can yield more information on exposure, as fewer subjects need to be studied. The case-control design therefore makes investigations based on large study populations more feasible, an important consideration since large studies are usually needed to reduce random error (see Chapter 8).

Perhaps the most frequently mentioned disadvantage of the case-control design is the difficulty in selecting a satisfactory control group, with the consequent problem of introducing systematic error in the study by the selection of controls. This problem is an issue only for non-random selection of controls. When the control group is defined as a random sample of the study population, control selection is a simple technical procedure and introduces no systematic error beyond what would be present in a cohort study using the entire study population. Using information from sample (controls) rather than from the entire study population does increase random variability (see the section on random error in Chapter 8), but when the size of the control group is adequate, this effect is small or negligible. The amount of random error that can be removed by expanding the control group to include the entire study population is often trivial, whereas the corresponding cost would be great.

In case-control studies involving contact with study subjects or their relatives, questions about previous exposure are usually answered by the study subjects only after the cases have fallen ill. The cases, therefore, may have spent more time thinking about past exposures and causes of their disease, while the controls have no motivation to do so. This difference between cases and controls in the accuracy and completeness of exposure information can introduce a "recall bias" into the study. A similar bias may be seen in cohort studies in which, for some reason, exposure information is obtained only after the cases have been identified.

When the induction period (time between exposure and disease appearance for the disease under study) is long, one or more decades may have to elapse between exposure and the beginning of the study observation period. This delay can often be avoided by collecting exposure information retrospectively in cohort studies as well as in case-control studies.

Study size

In epidemiologic investigations based on information from a small number of subjects there will be substantial random variation. There are statistical methods to estimate the study size required to produce reliable results in different situations (Greenland 1988).

A number of factors can influence the study size requirements, but in principle the number of cases, and in a case-control study, the number of controls, are the key factors in estimating the optimal study size.

The size of any study is usually limited by practical circumstances such as budget, time schedule or availability of cases. With a certain study population and observation period in mind, the investigator can use the study size as a basis for estimating hypothetical study results. A priori information is used to estimate the strength of the association (RR), as well as the occurrence of exposure and disease in the study population. These hypothetical results are then used to calculate the influence of random variation (e.g., 95 per cent confidence intervals) as described in Chapter 9. Should the level of random error turn out to be too high (i.e., the estimated confidence intervals are too wide), one should consider whether it would be meaningful to conduct a study of that size.

Additional Reading

Cornfield J: A Method of Estimating Comparative Rates from Clinical Data. Applications to Cancer of the Lung, Breast, and Cervix. Journal of the National Cancer Institute, 1951; 11: 1269–1275.

Doll R and Hill B: Mortality of British doctors in relation to smoking. Observations on coronary thrombosis; p. 205 in Haenszel W (ed): Epidemiological Approaches to the Study of Cancer and Other Chronic Diseases. National Cancer Institute; Monograph 19; US Department of Health, Education and Welfare, Public Health Service 1966.

Greenland S: On Sample Size and Power Calculations for Studies Using Confidence Intervals. American Journal of Epidemiology 1988; 128:231–237.

Haenszel W (ed): Epidemiological approaches to the study of cancer and other chronic diseases. National Cancer Institute, Monograph 19, US Department of Health, Education and Welfare, Public Health Service, 1966.

Mantel N and Haenszel W: Statistical aspects of the analysis of data from retrospective studies of disease. Journal of the National Cancer Institute 1959; 22:719–748.

McMichael AJ, Spirtas R, Kupper LL, Gamble JF: Solvent exposure and leucemia among rubber workers. Journal of the Society of Occupational Medicine 1975; 17:234–239.

Miettinen, OS: Matching and design efficiency in retrospective studies. American Journal of Epidemiology 1970; 91:111–118.

Miettinen OS: Estimability and estimation in case-referent studies. American Journal of Epidemiology 1976; 103:226–235.

Norell S: Principles of study design in epidemiology. Dept. of Epidemiology, Inst. of Environmental Medicine, Karolinska Institutet, Stockholm 1988.

Norell S, Ahlbom A, Erwald R et al: Diet and pancreatic cancer. A case-control study. American Journal of Epidemiology 1986; 124:894–902.

Norell S, Ahlbom A: Hospital vs. population referents in two case-referent studies. Scandinavian Journal of Work Environment and Health 1987; 13:62–66.

Olin R and Ahlbom A: The cancer mortality among Swedish chemists. Environmental Research 1980; 22:154–161.

8. Accuracy of Epidemiologic Studies

Validity and precision

An epidemiologic study may be considered a measurement of either the rate of occurrence of a disease or the effect of some exposure on the occurrence of a disease. As with other measurements the accuracy of the study result depends on "validity" and the "precision" of the measure.

Validity is the extent to which the study measures what it is intended to measure; lack of validity is referred to as "bias" or "systematic error." Precision is the reproducibility of a study result, that is, the degree of resemblance among study results, were the study to be repeated under similar circumstances: Lack of precision is referred to as "random error." The concepts validity and precision are often illustrated with the help of a target (see Figure 8.1). High validity corresponds to the average position of the shots being near the center. High precision corresponds to the shots being concentrated in a small area. A study that is based on information from too few subjects (usually too few exposed cases) allows for considerable random variation in the study result, since only a few extra cases occurring in one or another category would substantially affect the results. Such a study would have a low precision, with a corresponding wide confidence interval for the rate ratio (or rate difference - see Chapter 9).

The combination of high precision and a low validity is worth a comment on its own. The confidence in the result of a study is often considered to be greater if other studies show similar results, but such agreement can arise from precision that is unaccompanied by validity, if all the studies have a similar bias.

When evaluating a study it is essential to recognize that there will never be a study with perfect validity and precision. In assessing how accurate the result is, and in which direction is there most likely to be a bias, the reader will need information about the choice of study population and observation period, the methods that were used to identify the cases, the analytic techniques employed, and the precision of the study measures. The precision of a study result (e.g., the study estimate of RR) is stated by the confidence interval (see Chapter 9). If the investigation is a comparison of disease occurrence among exposed and unexposed, information is also needed about the methods used to divide people into exposed and unexposed groups and the methods used to control for the possible effect of other factors that could influence the occurrence of the disease under study. This information should be reported in such a way that the reader can form an intelligent opinion about the accuracy of the study.

Figure 8.1

Different combinations of high and low precision and validity

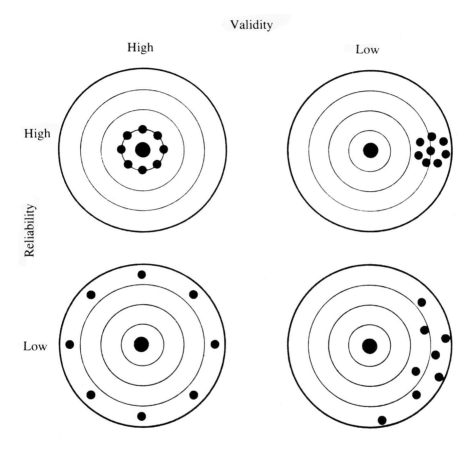

Validity in comparisons of disease occurrence

Epidemiologic studies generally are aimed at estimating the effect, if any, of some exposure on the occurrence of some disease. This evaluation is accomplished by contrasting the rates of disease occurrence among exposed and unexposed sub-populations. Systematic errors, leading to low validity, can arise in several different ways. The major sources of such errors are:

1. Confounding

The exposed and unexposed groups may differ with regard to the occurrence of some other factor or factors that influence the risk of developing the disease under study. If this difference is not taken into account, a systematic error generally referred to as "confounding" is introduced. For a more thorough discussion of "confounding" the reader is referred to the references given at the end of this chapter.

Example: In a study it was found that subjects with a high consumption of alcohol had a higher risk of developing lung cancer than those who did not drink alcohol. The reason for this association was that subjects with a high consumption of alcohol were often heavy smokers. Confounding from smoking explained the observed association between alcohol consumption and lung cancer.

Figure 8.2

The association between alcohol consumption and lung cancer—
an example of "confounding"

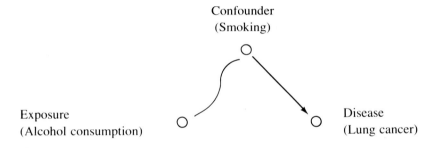

Confounder
(Smoking)

Exposure
(Alcohol consumption)

Disease
(Lung cancer)

2. Misclassification

The methods that are used to classify subjects with regard to exposure and disease, respectively, may introduce systematic errors in a study (misclassification). The extent of such misclassification depends upon the sensitivity and specificity of the method as well as on the relative frequency of the exposure and disease (Chapter 4). In addition, the effect of such misclassification depends upon whether it is "differential" or "non-differential." Exposure misclassification that is similar in sensitivity and specificity for those who develop the disease and those who do not, called "non-differential misclassification," results in a "diluting effect" that leads to an underestimation of the strength of the observed association. A similar error is introduced if the procedures used to identify cases of the disease under study have a low specificity that is similar for the exposed and unexposed. A more serious systematic error may be introduced if the misclassification for disease is different for the exposed and unexposed subjects, or if misclassification of exposure is different for cases and non-cases. Such "differential misclassification" may result in either an over- or underestimation of the observed association; the direction and magnitude of the bias may be difficult to evaluate (cf the discussion on recall bias in Chapter 7).

Example: The association between smoking and chronic bronchitis was investigated by comparing the disease occurrence for smokers and non-smokers. The possibility exists that smokers who have symptoms similar to those found in chronic bronchitis would be more likely than non-smokers to receive a diagnosis of chronic bronchitis, because the diagnostician might believe that smoking is associated with chronic bronchitis. This differential misclassification would adversely affect validity, leading to an overestimate of the effect of smoking on the occurrence of chronic bronchitis.

3. Selection bias

The selection of a particular study population and observation period may itself influence confounding and misclassification in epidemiologic studies. In case-control studies, the selection of controls may be an additional source of systematic error ("selection bias"). This bias is avoided if the controls are selected as a random sample of the study population (see Chapter 7, the section on case-control studies). Both in cohort studies as well as in case-control studies, exposed and unexposed subjects are followed up for disease occurrence during a certain period of time. A systematic error may be introduced if subjects are lost to follow-up. In case-control studies there is, in addition, the possibility that some of the cases identified and some of the controls selected may not be available for the collection of exposure information. Such non-response may also be a source of systematic error in the study.

Additional Reading

Greenland S, Robins JM: Confounding and misclassification. American Journal of Epidemiology 1985; 122:495–506.

Miettinen OS: Confounding and effect-modification: American Journal of Epidemiology 1974; 100:350–353.

Miettinen OS: Theoretical epidemiology: Principles of occurrence research in medicine. John Wiley & Sons, New York 1985.

Norell S: Principles of study design in epidemiology. Dept. of Epidemiology, Inst. of Environmental Medicine, Karolinska Institutet, Stockholm 1988.

Exercises—Chapters 7 and 8

1. Describe briefly the principles applicable to a

   a) cohort study.

   b) case-control study.

2. Give examples of situations where one should do a case-control study rather than a cohort study.

3. A case-control study gave the following results:

	Exposed	Unexposed
Cases	200	200
Controls	50	250

   Calculate the estimate of relative risk.

4. A case-control study of the association between smoking and myocardial infarction gave the following results:

	Non-smokers (unexposed)	Smokers (exposed) no. of packs/day		
		½	1	2
Cases	31	9	39	18
Controls	2,706	710	1,825	605

   Calculate the relative risk of myocardial infarction, with non-smokers as the reference group, for those smoking

   a) 1/2 pack per day

   b) 1 pack per day

   c) 2 packs per day

5. Of 595 patients who had received blood transfusions and 712 patients who had not, 75 and 16, respectively, developed hepatitis during a 2 1/2-year follow-up in a study designed to evaluate the relative risk.

   a) What is the type of study?

   b) Calculate the relative risk.

6. The incidence of myocardial infarction is higher in Finland than in Sweden. In the southern suburbs of Stockholm a study was conducted based on middle-aged men who developed myocardial infarction in the years 1974–76 and on controls from the general male population. Information was compiled on the country of origin and length of stay in Sweden.

	Finnish immigrants Number of years in Sweden		Swedes
	0–19	20+	
Cases	22	10	324
Controls	31	24	832

Calculate the relative risk of myocardial infarction among Finnish immigrants compared with Swedes.

a) for those living in Sweden for 0–19 years

b) for those living in Sweden for 20 years or more

7. In a case-control study 110 married women with myocardial infarction and 220 controls were interviewed. The questions were intended to identify women with hypertension, angina pectoris and diabetes, as well as to identify differences in education between husbands and wives. The results are shown in the table. Calculate the relative risk of developing myocardial infarction for women with

a) hypertension

b) angina pectoris

c) diabetes

d) an educational background that differs from that of her husband by more than one step on the scale.

	Cases		Controls	
	Exposed	Unexposed	Exposed	Unexposed
Hypertension	51	59	66	154
Angina pectoris	11	99	6	214
Diabetes	26	84	26	194
Education >1 step from husband's	19	91	14	206

8. To find out whether the use of oral contraceptives affects the risk of developing myocardial infarction, a case-control study was carried out among married nurses in the United States, where 159 hospitalized cases of infarction were compared with 3,180 controls. The results showed that 21 of the cases and 273 of the controls had used oral contraceptives.

a) Calculate the relative risk.

b) What potential confounders should be considered?

9. In a study of the association between acute non-lymphatic leukemia (ANLL) and occupational exposure to petroleum products the following procedure was employed: 50 consecutive cases of the disease were registered at a clinic and exposure to petroleum products was determined from occupational information. In the same way, 100 patients who had been treated for non-malignant complaints were registered and examined. The results are shown in the table below:

	ANLL	Non-malignant disease
Exposed	18	10
Unexposed	32	90
Total	50	100

a) What type of study is this?

b) Is there any association between the exposure studied and the disease?

c) Make a quantitative comparison of the disease occurrence between the exposed and unexposed groups.

d) In the absence of other details, can a possible association be interpreted as causal? Why or why not?

10. In a case-control study, interviews of cases and controls were conducted about diet, tobacco and alcohol habits that were suspected of being important for the development of the disease. The cases consisted of all the individuals in a defined population who during the course of one year had developed a certain form of cancer. What are the advantages or disadvantages in choosing the controls from among persons who during the year developed some other serious disease, instead of choosing controls from among healthy members of the population?

11. A case-control study is planned to investigate the association between alcohol consumption and myocardial infarction. Cases are chosen from the cardiology department of a university hospital. Two possible control groups have been suggested. One group comprises patients with injuries caused by accidents who arrive at the emergency department of the same hospital. The second control group comprises a representative sample from the population of the hospital's catchment area.

a) Which control group would give the greater relative risk?

b) What principal demand should be placed on the selection of a comparison group in this type of study?

c) Suggest a suitable control group bearing in mind (b), as well as the risk of drop-outs and differential misclassification of exposure.

12. What is meant by

   a) precision

   b) validity

13. Give your own example of

   a) confounding

   b) misclassification

   c) selection bias

14. The alcohol consumption of individuals in a random sample from a population was established. The individuals were divided into those who did and those who did not consume alcohol. A follow-up showed an excessive incidence of lung cancer among the consumers of alcohol. Discuss its validity.

15. In a case-control study individuals who have developed lung cancer and healthy controls are questioned about the occurrence of lung cancer among biological relatives. The aim is to study the impact of heredity on the occurrence of lung cancer.

   a) Discuss the possibility of differences in exposure misclassification between cases and controls.

   b) Name some conceivable confounding factors.

16. a) What conceivable confounding factors (apart from age) should be taken into account in a study of how work in a mine affects the incidence of lung cancer and cancer of the mouth and pharynx among men?

   b) What is required for these factors to be confounders?

17. The risk of a child being born with Down syndrome is known to increase with the mother's age. An investigation is planned to determine whether this risk is also influenced by the father's age.

   a) Name a confounding factor that should be borne in mind in the study.

   b) Why is this factor a confounder?

18. A study showed that women who drink at least five cups of coffee a day run double the risk (age-standardized RR) of others of developing

a myocardial infarction. A closer analysis showed, however, that this excess risk could almost completely be ascribed to one confounding factor. What is the confounder?

19. A cohort study is planned to investigate the association between the mother's alcohol consumption during pregnancy and Fetal Alcohol Syndrome in the new-born child. Discuss possible problems related to the identification of cases.

20. A case-control study of chronic lymphatic leukemia (CLL) showed that close relatives of the cases had the same disease considerably more often than expected. This finding might be interpreted as an expression of the importance of heredity for CLL. Suggest another interpretation.

21. Between 1949 and 1960 thousands of Israeli children received treatment with X-ray radiation (the equivalent of 120–140 rads at the surface of the brain hemispheres) for tinea capitis (scalp ringworm). To study if this X-ray radiation had affected the children's mental development, a follow-up was done of 11,000 exposed children. The results showed that they had lower IQs, poorer school reports and shorter education than a comparison group.

   a) Which possible confounding factors should one take into account if the comparison group was a representative sample of the population (of the same age and sex)?

   b) Make suggestions for choice of comparison group.

22. Persons who in their work have been exposed to asbestos are given health check-ups that include an X-ray examination of their lungs. Positive findings result in a more thorough examination in a hospital. At the outpatient department of a hospital, some investigators want to carry out a case-control study of X-ray-confirmed pleural plaques (pp) and occupational exposure to asbestos. Cases (with pp) and controls (without pp) represent all patients examined with X-ray at the department during one year. Discuss the validity.

23. A mass screening of a large number of middle-aged men included an examination of serum cholesterol. During a 3-year follow-up period mortality and causes of death were subsequently recorded. The men with low serum cholesterol (under 170 mg/100 ml) had significantly higher mortality from cancer than the others. Discuss the validity.

24. To find out whether the working environment and working conditions of firemen have an effect on the risk of dying from different diseases,

a comparison was made of the cause-specific mortality among 5,656 firemen in Boston with the corresponding mortality of the white male population of Massachusetts and the whole of the United States, respectively. The results showed an SMR less than 50% for mortality from infectious diseases, diabetes, rheumatic heart diseases, chronic nephritis, blood diseases and suicide. Discuss the validity.

25. In a survey it was found that alcohol consumption is negatively correlated with physical activity but positively correlated with smoking and obesity. Discuss the validity of a cohort study showing that consumers of alcohol have an increased risk of developing myocardial infarction.

26. A comparison showed that mothers who drink large amounts of alcohol during pregnancy give birth to children with a shorter length, lower weight, smaller head circumference and higher frequency of malformations than other children. What potential confounding factors should be taken into account if one wishes to draw conclusions about the effect of exposure to alcohol on the child's length, weight and head circumference as well as the risk of malformations?

27. Dietary habits, alcohol and tobacco consumption were studied in men with cancer of the larynx and a group of male controls. The results are shown in the following tables:

	Cases	Controls
Cigarette smoking (packs/day)		
0	43	163
$<\frac{1}{2}$	25	41
$\frac{1}{2}$–1	171	126
>1	135	51
Total	374	381
Alcohol consumption (units/month)		
0	38	87
<3	41	51
3–30	111	104
>30	179	116
Total	369	358
Vitamin A (IU/month)		
<50,500	98	78
50,500–150,500	201	216
>150,500	39	65
Total	338	359

Calculate the relative risk of cancer of the larynx:

a) at every level of cigarette smoking compared with non-smokers.

b) at every level of alcohol consumption compared with no alcohol consumption.

c) at every level of vitamin A consumption compared with the highest.

d) How should the results be interpreted?

e) What potential confounders should be expected in a study of the association between alcohol consumption and cancer of the larynx?

f) What should one bear in mind when selecting a control group in the study presented above?

28. Sketch a suggestion for an epidemiologic study to determine whether repeated exposure to X-rays has an effect on the risk of developing breast cancer. Discuss the validity.

29. Sketch a suggestion for an epidemiologic study to assess to what extent occupational exposure to wood dust has an effect on the risk of developing nasopharyngeal cancer. Discuss the validity.

9. Basic Principles of Data Analysis

Epidemiologic studies may be divided into two groups, according to their objectives. The first group comprises those studies in which the objective is simply to assess the occurrence of some disease in a certain population. The other comprises those studies in which the objective is to evaluate the association between an exposure and the occurrence of some disease. This chapter discusses the analyses of data from studies from each of these two groups. Analyses that take into account extraneous variables (variables other than disease and exposure) are deferred to the next chapter.

Measures of disease occurrence

In studies where the occurrence of disease is to be assessed, typically either the prevalence, cumulative incidence, or incidence rate is used as a measure of disease occurrence. The observed measure should be reported along with a "confidence interval" that provides some information as to the precision of the observed value. A confidence interval of 95%, say, is a range of values constructed to account for random variation in such a way that, if there were no systematic errors in the study, the probability that the interval would contain the "true" value is 95%. This means that, on the average, 95% of such intervals from valid studies would contain the true parameter value and that 5% would fail to do so. Thus, by assessing the confidence interval, information about the precision of the study is obtained. This assessment can be of great importance in epidemiologic studies where random variation stemming from a small number of diseased subjects plays an important role in interpretation. For a detailed discussion as to the calculation and interpretation of a confidence interval, the reader should refer to a textbook in statistics, e.g., Armitage (1971) or Colton (1974). See also the discussion in the next section of this chapter.

To calculate the confidence interval a probability model is needed; this model provides a means for calculating the probability of different possible study outcomes. In epidemiology the probability model called for is usually based upon either the "binomial distribution" or the "Poisson distribution." When the number of observations in a study is large, these models are often approximated by the "normal distribution" or "Gaussian" distribution, which leads to simpler formulas for calculating confidence intervals. The most important of these approximate formulas are the following:

a) Prevalence

Let the number of individuals with the disease be B and the total number of individuals in the population be N. According to the previous definition the prevalence is then

$$P = \frac{B}{N}$$

A 95% confidence interval is obtained as

$$P \pm 1.96 \sqrt{\frac{P(1-P)}{N}}$$

where the minus sign gives the lower limit and the plus sign the upper limit. The constant 1.96 corresponds to the desired 95% level of confidence. This confidence interval is based upon a normal distribution approximation of the binomial distribution.

Example: In an example in Chapter 2 reference was made to a study that assessed the prevalence of rheumatoid arthritis. In that study, B = 70 and N = 1,038, which gives P = 0.07. The 95% confidence interval would be:

$$0.07 \pm 1.96 \sqrt{\frac{0.07 \times 0.93}{1,038}} \quad \text{or } 0.05 - 0.09$$

b) Cumulative incidence

Let the number who become sick during the observation period be A and let the number of individuals at risk at the beginning of the period be N. We then have that:

$$CI = \frac{A}{N}$$

A 95% confidence interval is obtained according to the same principles as above since both the prevalence and the cumulative incidence are proportions:

$$CI \pm 1.96 \sqrt{\frac{CI(1-CI)}{N}}$$

Example: In another example in Chapter 2, it was mentioned that during a certain period 11 individuals out of 3,076 had developed brain tumors. Then A = 11, N = 3,076, and CI = 0.004. The confidence interval will be:

$$0.004 \pm 1.96 \sqrt{\frac{0.004 \times 0.996}{3,076}} \quad \text{or } 0.002 - 0.006$$

c) Incidence rate

If the number of cases that occur during the observation period is noted by A and the number of person-years by R, the incidence rate is:

$$I = \frac{A}{R}$$

The corresponding confidence interval is obtained as:

$$I \pm 1.96 \sqrt{\frac{I}{R}}$$

From the statistical point of view there is an important difference between the two previous measures and the incidence rate measure, since the former are proportions whereas the incidence rate is the ratio of the number of cases to the number of person years of experience. The basic probability model for incidence rates is the Poisson distribution. The confidence interval above is based on a normal distribution approximation of the Poisson distribution.

Example: In a third example in Chapter 2 the incidence rate for myocardial infarction was calculated. With the notation used here $A = 29$, $R = 41,532$, and consequently $I = 0.0007$. The confidence interval is calculated as follows:

$$0.0007 \pm 1.96 \sqrt{\frac{0.0007}{41,532}} \quad \text{or} \quad 0.0005 - 0.0010$$

Measures for comparison of disease occurrence

In contrast to studies that simply measure disease occurrence in a single group, studies of the association between an exposure and a disease compare the disease occurrence between subjects with different levels of exposure, as discussed in Chapter 5. Most often the rate ratio, or relative risk, defined as the ratio of the incidence rate in the exposed to that in the unexposed, is used. The ratio of cumulative incidence for exposed and unexposed groups may also be used. The comparison of disease occurrence need not be in the form of a ratio: it is also reasonable to estimate the difference in the rate of disease occurrence between the exposed and the unexposed groups. With systematic errors under control, any comparative measure of disease occurrence in populations with differing levels of exposure may be considered an effect measure.

Like simple measures of occurrence, effect measures should be presented along with an assessment of their precision. As before, precision is best described by the confidence interval.

The likelihood that the "true" value of a measure is located at a certain point within the confidence interval is not the same throughout the interval: the likelihood for the location of the point diminishes gradually towards the borders of the interval. Consequently, there is no sudden drop in likelihood at the boundaries of a confidence interval. For this reason, it is unwise to place too much attention on the exact location of the limits of the confidence interval. Furthermore, it should not be considered important if a certain value is or is not included within the confidence interval. Occasionally it is deemed essential for the interpretation of the results to determine whether the confidence interval includes or excludes the specific value that corresponds to no association between exposure and disease. That value is unity for the relative risk and zero for difference measures. This interpretation would be equivalent to performing a significance test of the hypothesis that there is no association. Because significance tests are less informative than confidence intervals and easily misinterpreted, we strongly recommend the use of confidence intervals in place of significance tests for assessing the precision in epidemiologic data. Furthermore, we would discourage the use of confidence intervals simply to determine whether the no-association value is included within the interval—that is, using the confidence interval as a surrogate for significance testing. For a further discussion of the interpretation of confidence intervals and significance tests, the reader can refer to articles by Poole (1987), Rothman (1978), and Walker (1986).

We shall describe the calculation of confidence intervals for the relative risk in some common epidemiologic situations. For a discussion of other situations, such as the use of difference measures, the reader should consult a comprehensive text (e.g., Rothman, 1986).

A general formula for the 95% confidence interval for the relative risk can be calculated as follows, if the number of observations is reasonably large so that the normal distribution approximation can be applied:

$$e^{\ln(RR) \pm 1.96\sqrt{\mathrm{var}[\ln(RR)]}}$$

(e is a mathematical constant approximately equal to 2.718, and ln is the logarithm function with e as base, the "natural" logarithm.) The exponent of e in this formula is the same kind of expression that was used in the previous section when confidence intervals were calculated around descriptive epidemiologic measures: It starts with the observed number, in this case ln(RR) (see below for a discussion about the role of the logarithm), and to this is added plus or minus 1.96 times the square root of the variance of the calculated number. This general formula for the confidence interval for RR is based on the normal distribution. Specific forms of this formula differ only in the variance calculation corresponding to the specific study design. The reason that the constant, e, and the natural logarithm are involved in the formula is that the distribution of possible values of the relative risk is highly asymmetric: the relative risk cannot be less than zero but has no upper limit. This asymmetry limits the applicability of the normal distribution, which is symmetric. The logarithmic transformation makes the distribution more symmetric, pulling in the long "tail" of large numbers and stretching the smaller tail toward negative infinity. The above formula for the confidence interval sets symmetric limits for a confidence interval on the logarithmic scale and then converts these limits back to the original scale by exponentiation. Below we give the specific formulas along with examples for some common epidemiologic situations.

Cohort studies—cumulative incidence:

In cohort studies where the cumulative incidence is used, data can be presented in a 2 × 2 table (see Table 9.1).

Table 9.1

Layout of the data from cohort study using cumulative incidence

		Exposed		
		Yes	No	All
Diseased	Yes	A_1	A_0	A
	No	N_1-A_1	N_0-A_0	$N-A$
	All	N_1	N_0	N

The relative risk is calculated as:

$$RR = \frac{A_1/N_1}{A_0/N_0}$$

and the variance of ln(RR) as:

$$var[\ln(RR)] = \frac{N_1 - A_1}{N_1 A_1} + \frac{N_0 - A_0}{N_0 A_0}$$

Based on this variance, the confidence interval can be calculated according to the formula given above.

Example: Assume that out of 100 exposed individuals 20 will develop a disease. In a comparison group of 200 unexposed individuals, 25 develop the disease. These data may be arranged in a 2 × 2 table (see Table 9.2).

Table 9.2

Number of individuals and cases in a cohort study, by exposure status

		Exposed		
		Yes	No	All
Diseased	Yes	20	25	45
	No	80	175	255
	All	100	200	300

The relative risk and the variance are calculated as:

$$RR = \frac{20/100}{25/200} = 1.60$$

$$var[\ln(RR)] = \frac{100 - 20}{100 \times 20} + \frac{200 - 25}{200 \times 25} = 0.0750$$

We therefore get the 95% confidence interval as:

$$e^{\ln(1.60) \pm 1.96\sqrt{0.0750}} = e^{-0.0668, \ 1.01} = 0.935, 2.74$$

Cohort studies—incidence rate:

In cohort studies where the number of person-years is available, the incidence rate will usually be the measure of choice. The analysis must take into account the distribution of person-years between the exposed and unexposed groups. Data may be arranged in a table like the one shown in Table 9.3.

Table 9.3

Layout of data from a cohort study using incidence rate

	Exposed		
	Yes	No	All
Cases	A_1	A_0	A
Person-Years	R_1	R_0	R

The relative risk is the ratio of the incidence rate in the exposed to that in the unexposed:

$$RR = \frac{A_1/R_1}{A_0/R_0}$$

With the incidence rate as the basis for the relative risk, the following variance formula is used:

$$var[\ln(RR)] = \frac{1}{A_1} + \frac{1}{A_0}$$

Example: In the previously referenced study of the association between smoking and mortality from coronary heart disease the following data were obtained:

Table 9.4

Number of cases and number of person-years in a cohort study by exposure status

	Cigarette smokers		
	Yes	No	All
Cases	206	28	234
Person-Years	28,612	5,710	34,322

Again we start with the calculation of the relative risk and the variance of the logarithm of the relative risk:

$$RR = \frac{206/28,612}{28/5,710} = 1.47$$

$$\text{var}[\ln(RR)] = \frac{1}{206} + \frac{1}{28} = 0.0406$$

The 95% confidence interval is now obtained as:

$$e^{\ln(1.47) \pm 1.96\sqrt{0.0406}} = e^{-0.0107, \ 0.778} = 0.989, \ 2.18$$

Cohort design—SMR

The SMR was defined in Chapter 5 as the ratio of the observed number of cases in a population, O, to a corresponding expected number, E. The data analysis is usually based on the assumption that the expected number is calculated on rates from such a large population that it can be considered a fixed number without any random inaccuracy. This assumption is often reasonable when the expected number is calculated from national or regional rates.

Given the assumption of a fixed expected number, a confidence interval is calculated around the observed number and the interval for the SMR is obtained by division with the expected number. For large numbers the confidence interval around the observed number is again based on a normal distribution approximation of the Poisson distribution and is calculated as:

$$O \pm 1.96\sqrt{O}$$

Example: Retrospective cohort studies were presented along with an example describing how to calculate the SMR. The example referred to a cohort consisting of chemical engineers. In the example we had $O = 32$ observed cases and $E = 24.2$ expected. We thus get the following confidence interval around the observed value:

$$32 \pm 1.96\sqrt{32} = 20.9, \ 43.1$$

By dividing each of these two confidence limits by the expected number of 24.2 we get $20.9/24.2 = 0.864, 43.1/24.2 = 1.78$ as the limits to a 95% confidence interval for the SMR.

Case-control design:

As has been seen before, case-control data may be arranged in a 2×2 table of the same kind as we used for cohort studies using cumulative incidence (see Table 9.5).

Table 9.5

Layout of data from a case-control study

	Exposed		
	Yes	No	All
Cases	a	b	N_1
Controls	c	d	N_0
All	a + c	b + d	N

The calculation of the confidence interval goes along the same lines as above: In case-control studies the relative risk is calculated as the odds-ratio:

$$RR = \frac{a/b}{c/d}$$

and the variance for the corresponding logarithm is taken as:

$$var[\ln(RR)] = \frac{1}{a} + \frac{1}{b} + \frac{1}{c} + \frac{1}{d}$$

Example: In a previous example data were presented from a case-control study on diet and pancreatic cancer. The data are shown in Table 9.6.

Table 9.6

Data from a case-control study on pancreatic cancer

	Grilled or fried meat weekly		
	Yes	No	All
Cases	53	43	96
Controls	53	85	138
Total	106	128	234

The relative risk and variance are:

$$RR = \frac{53/43}{53/85} = 1.98$$

$$var[\ln(RR)] = \frac{1}{53} + \frac{1}{43} + \frac{1}{53} + \frac{1}{85} = 0.0728$$

Thus, the confidence interval becomes:

$$e^{\ln(1.98) \pm 1.96\sqrt{0.0728}} = e^{0.153, \; 1.21} = 1.17, 3.35$$

It is worth noting that if the size of the control group were large, c and d would also be large, and if the control group were sufficiently large, the last two terms in the variance formula would vanish. In this situation the case-control study variance formula would be identical to the incidence rate cohort study variance formula. This comparison illustrates the principle discussed in Chapters 7 and 8 linking the cohort and the case-control study design: in the former the entire study population is used, but in the latter only a sample.

Additional Reading

Armitage P: Statistical methods in Medical Research. Blackwell Scientific Publishers, 1971.

Breslow NE & Day NE: Statistical methods in cancer research. Vol.1. The analysis of case-control studies. International Agency for Research on Cancer, 1980.

Breslow NE & Day NE: Statistical methods in cancer research. Vol.2. The analysis of cohort studies. International Agency for Research on Cancer, 1988.

Colton T: Statistics in medicine. Little, Brown and Company, 1974.

Rothman KJ: A show of confidence (editorial). New England Journal of Medicine 1978; 299:1362–1363.

Rothman KJ: Modern epidemiology. Little, Brown and Company, Boston, 1986.

Poole C: Beyond the confidence interval: American Journal of Public Health 1987; 77:195–199.

Walker AM: Reporting results of epidemiologic studies. American Journal of Public Health 1986; 76:556–558.

10. Stratified Data Analysis

Stratification is one way to study and control for the effects of variables other than exposure and disease in the data analysis. Stratification means that data are divided into subgroups, or strata. Stratification by gender or age, for example, means that the data are divided into categories of male and female or into categories of age. In Chapter 5 there was a section on standardization, in which age standardization was used as the example. Standardization is a procedure that exemplifies one type of stratified analysis.

The primary reason for conducting a stratified analysis is to evaluate and if necessary control for confounding. Confounding arises when some cause other than the exposure under study is more, or less, prevalent in the exposed group than in the unexposed. When data are stratified by levels of the confounding factor, for example in males and females, each stratum will be free from confounding from the stratification variable. That is, if the association between exposure and disease is analyzed separately in, say, males and females, each of the two strata of gender will give an estimate of the effect of exposure, free of confounding from gender. Often these stratum specific results are not reported separately, but pooled into a single result. This was the case in the age standardization example in Chapter 5, for instance, in which confounding by age was controlled.

Another reason to conduct a stratified analysis is the analysis of effect modification. Effect modification means that the effect of the exposure is stronger in some strata than in others. If, for example, the relative risk relating exposure and disease is 2 among females and 3 among males, gender would modify the effect of the exposure and, thus, be an effect modifier.

The basic principle for using stratification to control for confounding will be illustrated by means of two examples, one from a cohort study and another from a case-control study.

Cohort study

Table 10.1 displays the material from an epidemiologic study with a cohort design. The purpose of the study was to evaluate the association between alcohol consumption and a disease. There was a suspicion, however, that use of tobacco might be associated with the use of alcohol and also that tobacco itself could be a contributing cause of the disease. In other words, tobacco was considered a potential confounder in the study. For this reason, information was collected not only on use of alcohol but also on use of tobacco.

Table 10.1

Number of person years and number of cases by use of alcohol and by use of tobacco

Alcohol	Tobacco	Person-Years	Cases	I
No	No	75,000	75	0.001
No	Yes	25,000	50	0.002
Yes	No	25,000	50	0.002
Yes	Yes	75,000	300	0.004

If the information on tobacco use is disregarded the material can be described as in Table 10.2.

Table 10.2

Incidence rates by use of alcohol

Alcohol	I	RR
Yes	0.00350	2.8
No	0.00125	

The relative risk, obtained as the ratio of the incidence rate among exposed to that among unexposed, indicates a considerable association between alcohol and the disease. If, however, smoking is more common among those who use alcohol than among those who do not, and if, in addition, smoking is a cause of the disease, then the observed results could occur without alcohol use being causally related to the disease. (Recall the example on alcohol and lung cancer (Figure 8.2.) To examine this possibility, the data are stratified according to smoking. In this example, therefore, the data are divided into two strata, smokers and non-smokers. The stratified data are described in Table 10.3. The table shows that in both strata, i.e., for smokers as well as non-smokers, the incidence rate is two times as high for those who use alcohol as compared with those who do not.

Table 10.3

Incidence rates by use of alcohol and tobacco

Tobacco	Alcohol	I	RR
Yes	Yes	0.004	2
Yes	No	0.002	
No	Yes	0.002	2
No	No	0.001	

The relative risk decreased from 2.8 to 2.0 through the "control" of confounding from smoking. The estimate of 2.8 that was observed before smoking was

78

controlled can be thought of as reflecting a mixed effect of both alcohol and tobacco use.

A further analysis of the example shows that tobacco use fulfills the two criteria for confounding. From the column reporting the number of person-years in Table 10.1 it can be seen that there is an association between use of alcohol and use of tobacco. The table also reveals that tobacco in itself is associated with an increased incidence rate, both among the exposed (alcohol) and among the unexposed (no alcohol).

Note that although smoking is a confounder in the example shown in table 10.3, it is not an effect modifier; the relative risk is 2 both for smokers and for non-smokers.

Since strata often are small, the stratum specific relative risks tend to be shaky, that is their precision is often low. It is therefore desirable to pool the stratum-specific relative risks into one single, more stable relative risk. Pooling is reasonable if it appears unlikely, either from the data in hand or from *a priori* information, that the confounder is also an effect modifier.

In the above example the relative risk was 2 both for smokers and non-smokers, and therefore the pooled relative risk should also be 2. It is usually not the case, however, that the stratum-specific relative risks are identical. Hence, there is need for a formal procedure by which the pooling can be done. Such a procedure should take into account that some strata are more informative than others (because they have more data) and, thus, should receive more weight in the pooling process. Several such procedures are available. One is the Mantel-Haenszel technique, and another the maximum-likelihood technique. The maximum-likelihood technique is incorporated into popular multivariate methods such as the multivariate logistic regression model and the proportional hazards model. For a description of the maximum-likelihood techniques, the reader is referred to a more comprehensive textbook (e.g., Rothman 1986).

The relative risk pooled across strata according to the Mantel-Haenszel technique for cohort data based on incidence rates is calculated as (Rothman & Boice 1982):

$$RR = \frac{\Sigma A_1 R_0/R}{\Sigma A_0 R_1/R}$$

The summation is over all strata and $R = R_0 + R_1$. If cumulative incidence data were used instead, the number of person years would be replaced by the number of persons.

Example: The Mantel-Haenszel technique applied to the data in Table 10.1 gives:

$$RR = \frac{50 \times 75,000/100,000 + 300 \times 25,000/100,000}{75 \times 25,000/100,000 + 50 \times 75,000/100,000} = 2$$

That is, the Mantel-Haenszel relative risk equals the two stratum-specific values, as it should.

Pooled estimates of relative risk calculated for stratified data should be presented along with confidence intervals describing their precision. Confidence intervals for stratified data are calculated according to the same principles as were used in the previous chapter, but the variance formulas are more complex. In fact, reasonable variance formulas for the Mantel-Haenszel techniques were not presented until recently (Greenland & Robins 1985; Robins et al. 1986). These variance formulas are discussed in the text by Rothman (1986).

Case-control study

If all the cases and 200 controls are selected from the population that formed the basis of the previous example the following data should be expected.

Table 10.4

Number of cases and number of controls by use of alcohol and by use of tobacco

	Alcohol				
	Yes		No		
	Tobacco		Tobacco		
	Yes	No	Yes	No	All
Cases	300	50	50	75	475
Controls	75	25	25	75	200

Starting again by disregarding the information on tobacco use the data will be reduced to a 2 × 2 table:

Table 10.5

Number of cases and number of controls by use of alcohol

	Alcohol		
	Yes	No	All
Cases	350	125	475
Controls	100	100	200

The relative risk calculated from those numbers is:

$$RR = \frac{350 \times 100}{125 \times 100} = 2.8$$

After stratification for use of tobacco, we get instead the data shown in Table 10.6:

Table 10.6

Rate ratios associated with use of alcohol by use of tobacco

	Tobacco				
	Yes		No		
	Alcohol		Alcohol		
	Yes	No	Yes	No	All
Cases	300	50	50	75	475
Controls	75	25	25	75	200
RR		2		2	

In both strata of tobacco use the relative risk is estimated to be 2. Thus confounding will also occur in the case-control setting if use of tobacco is not controlled. The example also illustrates that, as in cohort studies, confounding in case-control studies can be controlled through stratification in the data analysis.

A pooled relative risk can be obtained for case-control data according to the same general principles as in the cohort study. The Mantel-Haenszel formula is:

$$RR = \frac{\Sigma ad/N}{\Sigma bc/N}$$

where again the summation is across all strata (Mantel-Haenszel 1959). The variance formula needed for the confidence interval calculation can be found in the same references as the cohort version (e.g., Rothman 1986).

Example: The data in Table 10.4 give the following Mantel-Haenszel relative risk:

$$RR = \frac{(300 \times 25)/450 + (50 \times 75)/225}{(50 \times 75)/450 + (75 \times 25)/225} = 2$$

Thus, the case-control study version of the Mantel-Haenszel relative risk formula also gives the expected result of 2.

Additional Reading

Breslow NE & Day NE: Statistical methods in cancer research. Vol.1. The analysis of case-control studies. International Agency for Research on Cancer, 1980.

Breslow NE & Day NE: Statistical methods in cancer research. Vol.2. The analysis of cohort studies. International Agency for Research on Cancer, 1988.

Greenland S & Robins JM: Estimation of a common effect parameter from sparse follow-up data. Biometrics 1985; 41:55–68.

Mantel N and Haenszel W: Statistical aspects of the analysis of data from retrospective studies of disease. Journal of the National Cancer Institute 1959; 22:719–748.

Robins JM, Greenland S & Breslow NE: A general estimator for the variance of the Mantel-Haenszel odds ratio. American Journal of Epidemiology 1986; 124:719–723.

Rothman KJ: Modern epidemiology. Little, Brown and Company, 1986.

Rothman KJ and Boice JD Jr.: Epidemiologic analysis with a programmable calculator. Epidemiology Resources Inc., 1982.

Exercises—Chapters 9 and 10

1. Calculate 95% confidence limits for the occurrence of hepatitis B markers in each of the two categories of personnel in exercise number 10 of Chapter 2. Describe the results in your own words.

2. Calculate 95% confidence limits for the occurrence of carcinoma in situ in exercise number 11 of Chapter 2.

3. Calculate 95% confidence limits for the occurrence of open angle glaucoma in exercise number 14 of Chapter 2.

4. Calculate 95% confidence intervals for the occurrence of bacterial meningitis in exercise number 15 of Chapter 2.

5. In exercise number 20 of Chapter 2 the occurrence of (a) stillbirth and (b) mortality among children born alive was calculated for children with a low birth weight. Calculate 95% confidence limits for (a) and (b), respectively.

6. Calculate 95% confidence limits for the occurrence of coronary heart disease in group (a) and group (d) in exercise number 22 of Chapter 2.

7. For exercise number 22, Chapter 2, calculate the relative risk for coronary heart disease in men with serum cholesterol 260 mg/10 ml and higher and systolic blood pressure 167 mm Hg and higher (group d) in relation to men with serum cholesterol under 220 mg/100 ml and systolic blood pressure under 147 mm Hg (group a). Calculate 95% confidence limits for the relative risk. Describe the results in your own words.

8. In exercise number 5, Chapter 7, patients who had and had not received blood transfusions were compared with regard to their risk of developing hepatitis. Calculate 95% confidence limits for the relative risk.

9. In exercise number 18, Chapter 2, the occurrence of injuries by moped accidents was compared between city and suburban inhabitants. Calculate the relative risk (city parish/suburb) for the age group 15–19 years. Calculate 95% confidence limits for the relative risk.

10. In exercise number 2, Chapter 6, the SMR was calculated for mortality from myocardial infarction among diabetics. Calculate 95% confidence limits.

11. In exercise number 4, Chapter 6, the SMR was calculated for malignant bone tumors among industrial workers exposed to radium. Calculate 95% confidence limits.

12. Calculate the relative risk of myocardial infarction for all smokers (1/2—2 packs of cigarettes per day) compared with non-smokers in exercise number 4, Chapter 7. Calculate 95% confidence limits.

13. In exercise number 6, Chapter 7, the relative risk of myocardial infarction was calculated for Finnish immigrants compared with native Swedes. Calculate 95% confidence limits for Finnish immigrants living in Sweden for

    a) 0–19 years

    b) 20 years or more

14. To study the effects of smoking and outdoor work (sun exposure) on the risk of developing cancer of the lip, a comparative study was made of men aged 50–69 years with cancer of the lip or skin. The results are shown in the table.

	Cancer of the	
	lip	skin
Smokers, outdoor work	51	6
Smokers, indoor work	24	10
Non-smokers, outdoor work	15	8
Non-smokers, indoor work	3	5

a) What is the design of this study?

b) Discuss the choice of reference group.

c) Calculate the relative risk of lip cancer for outdoor work compared with indoor work.

d) Calculate the stratum specific relative risks of lip cancer for outdoor work compared with indoor work after stratification for smoking and the Mantel-Haenszel relative risk.

e) Calculate the relative risk of lip cancer for smokers compared with non-smokers.

f) Calculate the stratum specific relative risks of lip cancer for smokers compared with non-smokers after stratification for work outdoors and indoors and the Mantel-Haenszel relative risk.

g) Calculate the relative risk of lip cancer for smokers with outdoor work compared with non-smokers with indoor work.

h) What is your interpretation of the results? How could the results have been affected by the choice of reference group?

Solutions to Exercises—Chapter 2

1. The population of the US increased during the period (from 117 to 230 million inhabitants). The mortality rate from cancer (number of cancer deaths in one year/100,000 inhabitants) increased by 61.5% from 1930 to 1970.

   The age distribution of the population has changed towards a greater proportion of older people. The age standardized mortality from cancer increased by 9.5% from 1930 to 1970.

   Improved diagnostic procedures may have contributed towards more deaths from cancer being recorded, but improved therapy may have contributed to a decrease in mortality from cancer.

2. Relative numbers. In comparisons of disease occurrence it is necessary to use measures that are independent of the size of the observed population.

3. Measures of incidence. These describe the flow from the disease-free state to the disease state, which is what one wishes to reduce through preventive measures.

4. a) 2% of the population have the disease at a specific point in time.
   b) Five cases of the disease occur per 10,000 person-years at risk.

5. The average duration of the disease decreases.

6. The incidence rate is the number of new cases of the disease that occur in relation to the risk period (disease-free years lived). The cumulative incidence is the number of individuals who get the disease during a period in relation to the number of individuals (free from disease) at the beginning of the period. The incidence rate, but not the cumulative incidence, is independent of the length of the observation period. The cumulative incidence is dimensionless and can only take on values from 0 to 1, while the incidence rate has the dimension "per unit of time" and can take on values from 0 with no upper limit.

7. Example 1: Of 100 individuals who were free of the disease at the beginning of the year, 90 developed a disease with very short (negligible) duration. Of these, 50 had the disease once, and 40, twice, during the year.

$$I = \frac{(50 \times 1) + (40 \times 2)}{100} = 1.3 \text{ per year}$$

$$CI = 90/100 = 0.9$$

While 90% of the individuals fell ill during the year, 1.3 cases of the disease occurred per person year at risk.

Example 2: Of 100 individuals who were free of the disease at the beginning of the year, 80 developed a long-term disease (duration more than $\frac{1}{2}$ year) after an average of six months.

Risk time = $(20 \times 1) + (80 \times \frac{1}{2})$ = 60 person-years
I = 80/60 = 1.3 per year
CI = 80/100 = 0.8 during one year

8. Number of cases = 532

Average size of population = $\dfrac{520 + 680}{2}$ = 600

Observation period = 4 years
Risk time = 600×4 = 2,400 person-years
I = 532/2,400 = 0.22 per year

9. P = 100/1,000 = 0.10

$CI = \dfrac{200}{1,000 - 100}$ = 0.22 over a 10-year period

Incidence cannot be calculated as the distribution of risk periods is unknown.

10. P_1 = 14/67 = 0.21
P_0 = 4/72 = 0.06

11. I = 123/338,294 = 0.00036 per year

12. P = 25/5,000 = 0.005

$CI = \dfrac{10}{5,000 - 25}$ = 0.002 over a 5-year period

13. Number of cases = 270

Average population size = $\dfrac{18,500 + 21,500}{2}$ = 20,000

Observation period = 5 years
Total risk period = $20,000 \times 5$ = 100,000 person-years
I = 270/100,000 = 0.0027 per year

14. P (cataract) = 310/2,477 = 0.125
P (senile macular degen.) = 156/2,477 = 0.063
P (diabetic retinopathy) = 67/2,477 = 0.027
P (open-angle glaucoma) = 64/2,477 = 0.026
P (blindness) = 22/2,477 = 0.009

15. I = $435/7,250,000 = 6.0 \times 10^{-5}$ per year

16. Number of cases = 97 + 121 + 112 = 330

$$\text{Avg. population size} = \frac{309,949 + 332,400}{2} = 321,174.5$$

Observation period $= 3$ years
Risk period $= 321,174.5 \times 3 = 963,523.5$ person-years
$I = 330/963,523.5 = 0.00034$ per year

17. $P_1 = 395/679,478 = 58 \times 10^{-5}$
    $P_2 = 0$

18. a) $I_1 = 21/80,000 = 26 \times 10^{-5}$ per year (suburb)
       $I_2 = 9/80,000 = 11 \times 10^{-5}$ per year (city parish)
    b) Age $= 15$–19 years:
       $I_1 = 20/4,000 = 500 \times 10^{-5}$ per year (suburb)
       $I_2 = 7/1,000 = 700 \times 10^{-5}$ per year (city parish)

    Age 20 years and over:
       $I_1 = 1/76,000 = 1.3 \times 10^{-5}$ per year (suburb)
       $I_2 = 2/79,000 = 2.5 \times 10^{-5}$ per year (city parish)

19. $P = 212/129,600 = 0.0016$

20. a) $P = 133/832 = 0.16$ (stillborn)
    b)

$$CI = \frac{210}{832 - 133} = 0.30 \quad \begin{array}{l}\text{(deaths during the first}\\ \text{month of life)}\end{array}$$

21. $P = 23,360/405,548 = 0.058$

22. a) $CI = 10/431 = 0.023$ over a 6-year period
    b) $CI = 19/185 = 0.103$ over a 6-year period
    c) $CI = 7/49 = 0.143$ over a 6-year period
    d) $CI = 11/44 = 0.250$ over a 6-year period

Solutions to Exercises—Chapters 3 and 4

1. Yes, through possible differences between the groups regarding the wording of the questions, the interviewer of the interview situation.

2. No, the agreement is not better than what one might have expected from chance alone:

Examiner A

		pos 0.1	neg 0.9
Examiner B	pos 0.1	0.01	
	neg 0.9		0.81

3. 1—The ophthalmologists' tendencies to make similar judgements.
    2—The number of categories (cup/disk ratios) which are used in the classification of findings.
    3—The distribution of the 100 examined optic disks between the different categories.

4. In the health screening material from routine gynecological check ups, one can expect a substantially smaller proportion with cervical cancer. This low prevalence places stringent demands on the method's specificity to avoid a substantial drop in the proportion of positives that are true positives (predictive value, see last section in chapter 4).

5. To exclude those individuals whose tests were carried out at laboratories B and C (alternatively stratify for lab).

6. Yes, differences in examination methods, diagnostic criteria and in the classification of diseases.

7. (Many examples can be given, but there are often certain variations—between different countries, hospitals and individual doctors—which can have significant consequences when measuring and comparing disease occurrence.)

8. a) The proportion of the sick classified as "sick."
    b) The proportion of the healthy classified as "healthy."

9. Sensitivity = 60/80 = 0.75
    Specificity = 80/120 = 0.67

10. Predictive value =

$$\frac{0.001 \times 0.99}{(0.001 \times 0.99) + (1 - 0.001) \times (1 - 0.99)} = 0.09 \ (9\%)$$

11. The test's sensitivity and specificity and the prevalence of the disease.

12. **P*/P**

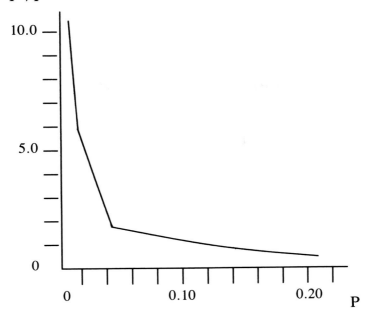

Solutions to Exercises—Chapters 5 and 6

1. Absolute   Relative

    I $60 - 15 = 45 \times 10^{-5}$ per year $60/15 = 4$

    CI $315 - 80 = 235 \times 10^{-5}$ during 5 yrs. $315/80 = 3.9$

    P $275 - 70 = 205 \times 10^{-5}$ $275/70 = 3.9$

2. $$\text{SMR} = \frac{1,107}{531} \times 100 = 208\%$$

   For diabetics the mortality due to myocardial infarction is 208% of—or about twice as big as—that of the whole population (after age standardization).

3. a) $CI_1 = 24/2,872 = 836 \times 10^{-5}$

      $CI_0 = 0$

      $$RR = \frac{CI_1}{CI_0} = \infty$$

   b) $CI_1 = 52/2,872 = 1811 \times 10^{-5}$

      $CI_0 = 6/5,055 = 119 \times 10^{-5}$

      $$RR = \frac{CI_1}{CI_0} = 15$$

   c) The relative risk for cancer of the thyroid cannot be estimated in a meaningful way since the comparison group was too small and/or the follow-up time too short for anyone to fall ill. There is, however, an appreciable difference between the groups (24 out of 2832 is considerably more than 0 out of 5055). Benign thyroid tumors were about 15 times more common in the exposed group.

4. $$\text{SMR} = \frac{22}{0.27} \times 100 = 8,148\%$$

   (i.e., mortality from bone tumors was about 80 times more common than for the population as a whole)

5. $$RR_{(b)} = \frac{CI(b)}{CI(a)} = \frac{19/185}{10/431} = 4.4$$

   $$RR_{(c)} = \frac{CI(c)}{CI(a)} = \frac{7/49}{10/431} = 6.2$$

   $$RR_{(d)} = \frac{CI(d)}{CI(a)} = \frac{11/44}{10/431} = 10.8$$

6. $\text{SMR} = \dfrac{11}{0.1} \times 100 = 11{,}000\%$

(The disease was about 110 times more common than expected).

7. a) $\text{CI}_1 = 3/95 = 316 \times 10^{-4}$
   $\text{CI}_0 = 8/48 = 1667 \times 10^{-4}$

   $\text{RR} = \dfrac{\text{CI}_1}{\text{CI}_0} = 0.19$

   b) $\text{RR} = \dfrac{0.27}{0.24} = 1.1$

   c) The occurrence of influenza among the vaccinated was about 20% of that of the placebo group (i.e., a decrease of 80%). The occurrence of discomfort after the "vaccination" was about 10% higher among those that had received the vaccine.

8. a) $\text{RR} = \dfrac{1.371}{1.228} = 1.1$

   b) $\text{RR} = \dfrac{498}{683} = 0.7$

   c) Mortality, but not morbidity, from myocardial infarction is lower among the married than among the unmarried. One possible interpretation is that the infarctions are milder (or receive better care) among the married.

9. Age-specific incidence rates:

	Group A	Group B
Younger	$4/2{,}000 = 0.002$	$20/4{,}000 = 0.005$
Older	$32/4{,}000 = 0.008$	$15/1{,}000 = 0.015$

   Age-standardized incidence rates (equal weights):
   Group A: $I_1 = (\tfrac{1}{2}) \times (0.002 + 0.008) = 0.005$
   Group B: $I_0 = (\tfrac{1}{2}) \times (0.005 + 0.015) = 0.010$

   $\text{RR} = \dfrac{I_1}{I_0} = 0.5$

10. $O = 40$

   $E = \dfrac{8{,}000 \times 0.5}{1000} + \dfrac{2{,}000 \times 4}{1000} + \dfrac{2{,}000 \times 9}{1000} = 30$

   $\text{SMR} = \dfrac{40}{30} \times 100 = 133\%$

11. $O = 8$

$$E = \left(\frac{651 \times 0}{337} + \frac{518 \times 6}{431} + \frac{500 \times 90}{522} + \frac{465 \times 381}{507} \right.$$
$$\left. + \frac{211 \times 626}{367} \right) \times 10^{-3} = 0.80$$

$$\text{SMR} = \frac{8}{0.80} \times 100 = 1,000\%$$

12. Age-standardized prevalence (equal weights):

$$P(I) = \frac{1}{4} \times \left(\frac{5}{1,000} + \frac{20}{2,000} + \frac{50}{4,000} + \frac{50}{3,000} \right) = 0.011$$

$$P(II) = \frac{1}{4} \times \left(\frac{25}{5,000} + \frac{40}{3,000} + \frac{20}{1,000} + \frac{20}{1,000} \right) = 0.015$$

$$\text{RR} = \frac{P(I)}{P(II)} = 0.7$$

13. Yes

PD $= 8 + 14 = 22\%$

CPD $= 29 + 14 = 43\%$

With no correlation between PD and CPD, $0.22 \times 0.43 = 0.09$; i.e., 9% would have both PD and CPD.

One possible explanation is that CPD can cause PD; another is that CPD and PD have the same causes in certain cases.

14. a) (see first two sections of chapter 6, pp 36–38)

b) Knowledge of risk indicators can be used to identify high risk groups, while knowledge of contributing causes also suggests what should be changed in order to prevent the disease.

15. a) Tubercle bacillus

b) Necessary cause

16. (See second section of chapter 6, pp 37–38)

17. a) 40%—100%

b) RR > 1

18. (See third section of chapter 5, pp 33–34 and last section of chapter 6, pp 38–40)

19. (See last section of chapter 6, pp 38–40)

20. $0.1 \times 0.2 \times 0.3 = 0.006$

21. a) 0.018
     0.012
     0.066
    b) 4
       3
       12
    c) The effect of increasing both B and C simultaneously is greater than the sum of the effects obtained if B and C are increased separately (see last part of the last section in chapter 6, p 40).

22. The occurrence among the population of that contributing cause. The occurrence of the other contributing causes in the same sufficient cause (see last section of chapter 6, p 40).

Solutions to Exercises—Chapters 7 and 8

1. (See chapter 7, e.g., Figures 7.1 and 7.2)

2. For example, in the event of rare diseases. (See chapter 7.)

3.
$$RR = \frac{200 \times 250}{100 \times 50} = 10$$

4. a)
$$RR = \frac{9 \times 2,706}{31 \times 710} = 1.1$$

   b)
$$RR = \frac{39 \times 2,706}{31 \times 1,825} = 1.9$$

   c)
$$RR = \frac{18 \times 2,706}{31 \times 605} = 2.6$$

5. a) Cohort study
   b)
$$RR = \frac{75/595}{16/712} = 5.6$$

6. a)
$$RR = \frac{22 \times 832}{31 \times 324} = 1.8$$

   b)
$$RR = \frac{10 \times 832}{24 \times 324} = 1.1$$

7. a)
$$RR = \frac{51 \times 154}{59 \times 66} = 2.0$$

   b)
$$RR = \frac{11 \times 214}{99 \times 6} = 4.0$$

   c)
$$RR = \frac{26 \times 194}{84 \times 26} = 2.3$$

   d)
$$RR = \frac{19 \times 206}{91 \times 14} = 3.1$$

8. a)
$$RR = \frac{21 \times 2,907}{138 \times 273} = 1.6$$

   b) Age, smoking, overweight, history of hypertension and other factors that may be correlated to the use of oral contraceptives and affect the risk of myocardial infarction.

9. a) Case-control study
   b) Yes
   c)
$$RR = \frac{18 \times 90}{32 \times 10} = 5.1$$

   d) No, possible validity problems must be taken into account.

10. Advantages: Perhaps less non-response and less difference between the groups in the quality of data (see chapter 7).

    Disadvantages: The possibility that the control group does not reflect the occurrence of the exposure in the population from which the cases were recruited.

11. a) The population sample
    b) The control group should be selected so that it reflects the presence of exposure in the population from which the cases are recruited.
    c) A group of patients whose disease (as opposed to injuries caused by accidents) is not correlated to alcohol consumption.

12. (See first section of chapter 8.)

13. (Consult the examples in chapter 8.)

14. Smoking is likely to be a confounder.

15. a) Compared to a healthy control, a person with lung cancer is perhaps considerably more aware of cases of lung cancer that have occurred in his family. This source of error is probably of less importance for close relatives (parents, brothers and sisters) than for more distant relatives.
    b) Smoking, radon radiation in homes and other factors that may vary in correlation to the "exposure" (biological relationship with someone who has had lung cancer) and affect the lung cancer risk.

16. a) Alcohol (cancer of the mouth and pharynx), radon radiation in homes (lung cancer), smoking (both) and other factors that may vary in correlation to the exposure (mining work) and affect the risk of the respective type of cancer.
    b) That they are unequally distributed in the two groups (exposed and unexposed, respectively) and that they affect the risk of developing the respective type of cancer.

17. a) Mother's age
    b) The mother's age varies in correlation to the studied "exposure" (= father's age) and affects the risk of Down syndrome.

18. Smoking

19. The diagnosis of "Fetal Alcohol Syndrome" is probably affected by knowledge of exposure, i.e., alcohol consumption during pregnancy.

20. Close relatives may be "exposed" to similar environmental factors or living habits. These may affect the risk of developing CLL.

21. a) Social background, heredity and other factors that may vary in correlation to the exposure (X-ray treatment for tinea capitis) and affect school reports, etc.

b) Brothers and sisters of the exposed children, or possibly the same as (a) but, in addition, with similar social and ethnic background.

22. Selection bias. X-ray examination of the lungs and detection of pleural plaques come about through the health check-ups to a greater degree among those exposed to asbestos than among those who are not so exposed.

23. Confounding. A cancer—detected or undetected—can cause both low serum cholesterol and death from cancer within 3 years.

24. Probably so-called healthy worker effect (see chapter 7).

25. Confounding.

26. Tobacco, medicines and infections during pregnancy, nutrition (mother's dietary habits), social background, heredity and possibly other factors that may conceivably vary in correlation to the exposure (alcohol during pregnancy) and affect the risk of small weight, height, etc., and of malformations.

27. a) 0 pk/day $\qquad$ RR $= 1.0$

    $<\frac{1}{2}$ pk/day $\qquad$ RR $= \dfrac{25 \times 163}{43 \times 41} = 2.3$

    $\frac{1}{2}$–1 pk/day $\qquad$ RR $= \dfrac{171 \times 163}{43 \times 126} = 5.1$

    >1 pk/day $\qquad$ RR $= \dfrac{135 \times 163}{43 \times 51} = 10.0$

  b) 0 unit/month $\qquad$ RR $= 1.0$

    <3 unit/month $\qquad$ RR $= \dfrac{41 \times 87}{38 \times 51} = 1.8$

    3–30 unit/month $\qquad$ RR $= \dfrac{111 \times 87}{38 \times 104} = 2.4$

    >30 unit/month $\qquad$ RR $= \dfrac{179 \times 87}{38 \times 116} = 3.5$

  c) $>150,500$ IU/month $\qquad$ RR $= 1.0$

    50,500–150,500 IU/month $\qquad$ RR $= \dfrac{201 \times 65}{39 \times 216} = 1.6$

    $<50,500$ IU/month $\qquad$ RR $= \dfrac{98 \times 65}{39 \times 78} = 2.1$

  d) There is an association (with "dose-response" relation) between cancer of the larynx and the consumption of tobacco, alcohol and vitamin A, respectively. Data provide, however, no information about how these consumption habits are related to one another and possible other "exposures" (confounding?) or how the groups were selected and the exposure measured (selection or information bias?)

e) Tobacco, vitamin A and other factors that may vary in correlation to the alcohol consumption and affect the risk of cancer of the larynx.

f) That the control group should reflect the consumption of tobacco, alcohol and vitamin A in the population from which the cases come. That the non-response can be kept at a low level and that the data quality at the measuring of the exposure can be similar to that for the cases.

28. Example of study: of the women with tuberculosis who had been discharged from two sanitoria during a certain period (1930–54), some (n_1 = 1,042) had received a treatment that included a large number of examinations with pulmonary X-ray (on average 100 per person) while the remaining women (n_2 = 722) had received another treatment. For each of the two groups a comparison was made of the number of observed cases of mammary cancer after discharge with the expected number on the basis of the occurrence of the disease in the female population (indirect age standardization). The results are shown in the following table:

	Observed number of cases	Expected number of cases
Exposed groups (n_1 = 1,042)	41	23.3
Unexposed groups (n_2 = 722)	15	14.1

A possible validity problem in studies where the exposure is a medical treatment of examination (for example pulmonary X-ray), is that the disease that is treated or examined (e.g., TB) can in itself be a risk indicator for the disease studied (e.g., mammary cancer). In the present example identification has been made of two groups of women with TB, one of which has been exposed to a large number of examinations with pulmonary X-ray.

29. (Different possibilities exist. The validity problems depend upon the design.)

Solutions to Exercises—Chapters 9 and 10

1.
$$P_1 = 0.21 \pm 1.96 \sqrt{\left(\frac{0.21\,(1 - 0.21)}{67}\right)} = 0.21 \pm 0.10$$

Among the personnel of wards with carriers, the proportion with hepatitis B markers is 11–31% (with 95% confidence).

$$P_0 = 0.06 \pm 1.96 \sqrt{\left(\frac{0.06\,(1 - 0.06)}{72}\right)} = 0.06 \pm 0.05$$

Among other personnel, the proportion with hepatitis B markers is 1–11% (with 95% confidence).

2.
$$I = 0.00036 \pm 1.96 \sqrt{\left(\frac{0.00036}{338,294}\right)} = \begin{array}{c} 0.00036 \pm 0.00006 \\ \text{per year} \end{array}$$

3.
$$P = 0.026 \pm 1.96 \sqrt{\left(\frac{0.026\,(1 - 0.026)}{2,477}\right)} = 0.0026 \pm 0.006$$

4.
$$I = 6.0 \times 10^{-5} \pm 1.96 \sqrt{\left(\frac{0.00006}{7,250,000}\right)} = \begin{array}{c} (6.0 \pm 0.6) \times 10^{-5} \\ \text{per year} \end{array}$$

5. a)
$$P = 0.16 \pm 1.96 \sqrt{\left(\frac{0.16\,(1 - 0.16)}{832}\right)} = 0.16 \pm 0.02$$

b)
$$CI = 0.30 \pm 1.96 \sqrt{\left(\frac{0.30\,(1 - 0.30)}{699}\right)} = 0.30 \pm 0.03$$

6.
$$CI(a) = 0.023 \pm 1.96 \sqrt{\left(\frac{0.023\,(1 - 0.023)}{431}\right)} = 0.023 \pm 0.014$$

during 6 years.

$$CI(d) = 0.250 \pm 1.96 \sqrt{\left(\frac{0.250\,(1 - 0.250)}{44}\right)} = 0.250 \pm 0.128$$

during 6 years.

7.
$$RR = \frac{11/44}{10/431} = 10.8$$

$$\exp\left[\ln(10.8) \pm 1.96\sqrt{\left(\frac{44-11}{44 \times 11} + \frac{431-10}{431 \times 10}\right)}\right]$$
$$= \exp(1.58, 3.18) = 4.85, 23.9$$

8. $$RR = \frac{75/595}{16/712} = 5.61$$

$$\exp\left[\ln(5.61) \pm 1.96\sqrt{\left(\frac{595-75}{595 \times 75} + \frac{712-16}{712 \times 16}\right)}\right]$$
$$= \exp(1.20, 2.25) = 3.31, 9.52$$

9. $$RR = \frac{7/1000}{20/4000} = 1.40$$

$$\exp\left[\ln(1.40) \pm 1.96\sqrt{\left(\frac{1}{7} + \frac{1}{20}\right)}\right]$$
$$= \exp(-0.524, 1.20) = 0.592, 3.31$$

10. $SMR = 1107/531 = 2.08$ (expressed as a ratio, not as a percentage)
$$1107 \pm 1.96\sqrt{1107} = 1041, 1172$$
$$1041/531 = 1.96, \quad 1172/531 = 2.21$$

11. $SMR = 22/0.27 = 81.5$ (expressed as a ratio, not as a percentage)
$$22 \pm 1.96\sqrt{22} = 12.8, 31.2$$
$$12.8/0.27 = 47.4, \quad 31.2/0.27 = 116$$

12. $$RR = \frac{66 \times 2706}{31 \times 3140} = 1.83$$
$$\exp[\ln(1.83) \pm 1.96\sqrt{(1/66 + 1/2706 + 1/31 + 1/3140)}]$$
$$= \exp(0.174, 1.04) = 1.19, 2.82$$

13. a) $$RR = \frac{22 \times 832}{31 \times 324} = 1.82$$
$$\exp[\ln(1.82) \pm 1.96\sqrt{(1/22 + 1/832 + 1/31 + 1/324)}]$$
$$= \exp(0.0389, 1.16) = 1.04, 3.19$$

b)
$$RR = \frac{10 \times 832}{24 \times 324} = 1.07$$

$$\exp [\ln (1.07) \pm 1.96\sqrt{(1/10 + 1/832 + 1/24 + 1/324)}]$$
$$= \exp (-0.681, 0.816) = 0.506, 2.26$$

14. a) Case-control study.

b) The control group should reflect the occurrence of the exposure in the population. This is not the case if, for example, skin cancer is more common in people who work outdoors.

c)
$$RR = \frac{(51 + 15) (10 + 5)}{(24 + 3) (6 + 8)} = 2.62$$

d)
$$RR \text{ (smoke)} = \frac{51 \times 10}{24 \times 6} = 3.54$$

$$RR \text{ (no smoke)} = \frac{15 \times 5}{8 \times 3} = 3.13$$

$$RR_{M-H} = \frac{(51 \times 10)/91 + (51 \times 5)/31}{(6 \times 24)/91 + (8 \times 3)/31} = 3.40$$

e)
$$RR = \frac{(51 + 24) (8 + 5)}{(15 + 3) (6 + 10)} = 3.39$$

f)
$$RR \text{ (out)} = \frac{51 \times 8}{6 \times 15} = 4.53$$

$$RR \text{ (in)} = \frac{24 \times 5}{10 \times 3} = 4.00$$

$$RR_{M-H} = \frac{(51 \times 8)/80 + (24 \times 5)/42}{(15 \times 6)/80 + (3 \times 10)/42} = 4.33$$

g)
$$RR = \frac{51 \times 5}{6 \times 3} = 14.2$$

h) The results (d and f) indicate that the risk of lip cancer is increased both by outdoor work and by smoking. Without stratification (c and e) the relative risks are somewhat underestimated. This is due to a correlation between smoking and indoor work. The combined effect of smoking and outdoor work (g) seems to be more than additive.

If outdoor work increases the risk of skin cancer (control group), this would result in an underestimation of the relative risk of lip cancer in outdoor work.

Index